With a Little Help
from Our Friends

With a Little Help from Our Friends
Creating Community as We Grow Older

☙☙

BETH BAKER

Vanderbilt University Press

Nashville

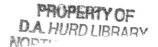

This book is the recipient of the
Norman L. and Roselea J. Goldberg Prize
from Vanderbilt University Press
for the best project in the area of medicine.

This book is printed on acid-free paper.
Manufactured in the United States of America

Library of Congress Cataloging-in-Publication Data on file
LC control number 2013041118
LC classification number RA564.8.B345 2014
Dewey class number 362.16—dc23

ISBN 978-0-8265-1987-0 (cloth)
ISBN 978-0-8265-1988-7 (paperback)
ISBN 978-0-8265-1989-4 (ebook)

To Ross

for his support in so many ways

Contents

Acknowledgments

This book would not have been possible without the openness of the many people who allowed me to visit their communities and who were willing to share their stories. Their names are in these pages, and I thank each one of them for their time, their honesty, and their trust. In particular, Gail Kohn was a valuable resource and font of insights who made many of these journeys more rewarding (and fun). My friend Barbara Armstrong greatly encouraged me with her enthusiastic review of my manuscript. Katie Pugliese contributed her considerable computer skills to assist me with the index. My wonderful neighbors and the members of the Washington Ethical Society have taught me the meaning and value of living surrounded by a close community of support. Many other friends and family members—you know who you are—have consistently believed in this project and encouraged me throughout the years I worked on it. Finally, Michael Ames, director and editor of Vanderbilt University Press, has been a steadfast believer in my work, and for that I am eternally grateful.

With a Little Help from Our Friends

Prologue
The Oncoming Train

In 1922, my maternal great-grandfather Albert Nisley and my great-aunt Marie were killed by a train after their car stalled on the railroad tracks. From the time I was a little girl, I wondered how this could have happened. Why did they not get out of the car in time? I picture my great-grandfather desperately trying to start the engine. Did he shout at his daughter to escape while she could? Did she refuse to abandon him? Were they on a blind curve and did not realize that disaster loomed?

My mother, who was three years old at the time, could not answer these questions. "It wasn't that uncommon," she shrugged. "You heard about accidents like this. Maybe they didn't know how fast the train was coming."

The scene of this drama was outside of Washington Courthouse, Ohio, a rural community thirty-five miles southwest of Columbus where my mother was born and raised. It still looks much the same, flat land broken by the occasional grove of trees and neatly kept farmhouses, barns, and silos. Farmers on enormous combines now cultivate hundreds of acres of corn and soybeans, and the small farms have given way to ever larger holdings.

The train wreck changed the lives of my grandparents, Ralph and Elsa, in unwelcome ways. Good, upright Methodists with a strong moral compass, they accepted the heavy mantle of duty. At the time, they lived in the small house down the road from the family farm, where my cousins still live. My grandparents were contented there. But when my great-grandfather was killed, all that changed. My great-grandmother Hannah expected my grandparents to move into the main farmhouse and take care of it and of her.

Elsa did her duty, but I can picture her, lips pursed, doing her chores with resentment. Her brother-in-law and his wife, she believed, could have moved in with Hannah, with whom Elsa did not get along. After all, they did not have children, while my grandmother had two little girls to care for, with another to come soon after.

To make matters more difficult, my great-grandmother may have developed Alzheimer's disease or some other type of dementia. "I remember she asked me once, 'Did you ever darn ears?'" my mother told me, laughing and still mystified. Such an odd question that it stayed with her for more than eighty years. Toward the end of her life, my great-grandmother stayed upstairs in her room, tended by a nurse. When she died, the funeral was held there in the farmhouse parlor.

Because of this story, I have always been a bit skeptical about the good old days when families took care of their own. Much as we like to think of those times wrapped in a rosy gauze of nostalgia, the truth was often more complicated. Friction and misunderstandings are as old as human families.

Nevertheless, throughout history, and still today in many cultures, families were expected to care for their elders. Midway through the twentieth century, this narrative shifted in the United States. Along with the death of the family farm, the outward migration to far-flung places for work and women entering the workforce in greater numbers led to the unraveling of the old rules and assumptions.

A dominant refrain of the older generation became, "I don't want to be a burden on my children," and an often unspoken corollary, "I want to stay independent; I don't want my children to control my life."

But this new perspective on aging may be no more satisfying than the old obligations of extended family. After my father died, my mother kept their house for many years but eventually moved to a continuing care retirement community, first living independently, then in assisted living, and finally dying in the rehab section of the nursing home. It was not a future I would want for myself.

Although she had a lovely small apartment in assisted living, a sense of ownership and control is difficult to maintain once you are in a large facility. Many forces conspire to undermine your autonomy, and in small ways you are made aware that you are a visitor and not the mistress of your castle. My mother had all of her faculties, including her Scrabble skills and wonderful wit. Yet because of institutional fire concerns, she was not allowed to have a toaster. I feel a deep dread as I imagine myself in that situation, a fear of that loss of control. Of course my mother could have wheeled herself down to the dining room and gotten whatever breakfast she wanted. But she was a late riser and liked to have a leisurely breakfast in her robe. The price she paid, then, was to spend her final year beginning each day with a wistful longing for hot buttered toast.

My mother-in-law would seem to have it better. At age ninety-five, though frail with multiple mild medical problems, Ruth lives in a roomy apartment in a high-rise complex where she and my father-in-law moved nearly thirty years ago in downtown Silver Spring, a suburb of Washington, DC. She is fiercely independent and would not dream of moving to an age-restricted community as my mother did. While my mother had an almost Zen-like detachment from her "stuff," Ruth is surrounded by a wealth of belongings that are precious to her: hundreds of books and videos; her mother's gold embossed china; her piano, which she plays regularly; family photos; file drawers of articles and leaflets from political and union organizing; and art work that covers every available inch of walls. Only in the last few years did she hire someone to help with cleaning once a month.

But even with the blessings of independence, my mother-in-law faces difficulties. She no longer drives, and as she has grown more frail, she finds it more difficult to use public transportation. She is lonely and misses not only the companionship of her husband of fifty-two years, but also of friends who have died or moved away. She spends considerable time going to doctor appointments. She clings to the silver thread of hope that nothing will happen to her physically or mentally to unravel her present situation. Meanwhile her rent has escalated dramatically, and she wonders if her fixed income and savings will be enough to allow her to remain where she is.

My family, then, represents the range of options that have existed for most people in our country as they age: move in with family, move to a retirement community or long-term care, or live alone.

But these are not the only ways we can imagine growing old. A significant cultural shift is underway. More than any other time in human history, people of the "Third Age" are realizing that they can make other choices about where and how to live. With intention and planning, people around the nation are creating ways to live in community, alternatives that give them more control, more companionship, more dignity and choice than generations past.

In my last book, *Old Age in a New Age*, I told the story of a movement dedicated to transforming nursing homes, those institutions of last resort, to homey communities based on relationships and person-centered living. What drew me to that topic were the inspiring leaders who were committed to sweeping transformation. I learned that with imagination, commitment, and hard work, people can find solutions to seemingly intractable problems.

This book, too, is a story of imagination, commitment, and hard work. But unlike the culture change movement in long-term care, this movement is driven less by enlightened organizations than by small groups of individuals—families, friends, neighbors, or kindred spirits—bonding together to take charge of their destiny as best they can.

As I enter my sixties, my own perspective on growing old is evolving. The aftermath of my great-grandfather's fatal crash continues to ripple, affecting me four generations later. I don't want to be caught unawares, oblivious to the oncoming train. Neither do I want to be the survivor, like my grandmother, who feels she has no choices. It's time for my generation to slow down, see what's around the bend, and choose wisely.

PART I

A Time Like No Other

CHAPTER 1

The End of Denial
Taking Charge of How We Live

Lynne, a fifty-something dietician in Port Gibson, Mississippi, has had a fantasy for years. When she grows older, rather than move to a retirement community or live alone, she and a handful of close friends will find a way to be together. "We talked about buying a piece of property and building us a place to live," she said. "We envisioned maybe a round building, where everyone had their own apartment, to come and go as they please, but also a central living area. We would be some place we had chosen as a group. We would hire someone to cook and clean for us. That would be a way of taking care of each other, but still have privacy."

Conversations like this are happening all over the United States, as my generation of baby boomers realizes that middle age will soon be in the rearview mirror. And then what?

That question often arises as we struggle to assist our parents, now very old, as they lose mobility, lose memory, lose independence. We see them, whether resistant or acquiescent, cheerfully accepting or refusing "to go gentle," and it is troubling, even terrifying, to imagine ourselves in their shoes. Can it really be that in a blink of an eye we will be the ones our own children fret about? Will we face the same limited choices as our parents?

And will we continue the age-old practice of denial? The SCAN Foundation, which focuses on transforming health care, including long-term care, in ways that foster independence, dignity, and choice as we grow older, has held focus groups around the country of people who are forty to sixty-five years old and who have been family caregivers. What these conversations revealed was that participants of all ethnic and class backgrounds were unable to imagine themselves as growing frail and needing help. "They can describe the experience of caregiving very accurately," said foundation CEO Bruce Chernof,

---

Unless otherwise indicated through a note, all quotes come from my interviews, whether in person, over the telephone, or through email. To protect people's identities I use their first names, except in cases where the individuals are already publicly known. In a few cases, I use a fictitious name at the request of the interviewees.

MD, in an interview. "People acknowledge it was a lot of work. Generally people were caring for someone who was a family member or close friend and they felt a lot of pride in what they had done. Even though they could intellectually describe it, when they applied that knowledge to themselves, they couldn't do it." It's almost as if we are hard-wired to not imagine our own vulnerability.

Many of us have said our last good-byes to parents, and suddenly, there at family gatherings and funerals, we turn around and realize to our surprise we *are* the old ones. The torch is ours, whether or not we are ready to accept it.

"The very cultural and technological forces that protect us from early death are also redrawing the social maps we need to find our way through life," wrote geriatrician William H. (Bill) Thomas, MD, a pioneer in transformative eldercare. "Long-settled ideas about how life is to be lived are remade in less than a lifetime."[1]

Our nation and indeed the world are undergoing unprecedented demographic change. In 1900, 4 percent of Americans were over sixty-five. Today that figure is 13 percent; it will be 17 percent by 2020 and continue to grow over the next twenty years or more, fueled by seventy-two million baby boomers. "Those may not seem like big differences, but they're huge," said Margaret Perkinson, a gerontological researcher at St. Louis University.

Throughout human history, cultures have taken a similar trajectory, she explained. Preindustrial societies have a high birth rate and a high death rate. People die from infectious diseases, poor sanitation, and lack of food. In the next stage people start to live longer but the birth rate is still high, with families counting on children to help in the fields. "With improvements in public health, you tend to have a population still relatively young, but increasing in size," she said. "In the next stage, the birth rate starts to decline because you get to a point where there are a lot of cultural changes, shifting from an agricultural to an industrial economy, where it's no longer as advantageous to have huge families." Labor laws prohibit children working in factories, and as women join the workforce, caring for large families becomes expensive and difficult. With both a declining birth rate and a declining death rate, the population grows relatively older.

These sweeping changes have very real consequences for individuals and families, said Perkinson. As recently as 1900, the average US life expectancy was just forty-five (in part due to high infant mortality, not only to people dying at a younger age). "The demands of caring for older adults are much more significant than they were before," she said. "In the past, in a typical family, the father would die before the children left home. The whole notion of empty nest is a modern concept. The notion of retirement is a modern concept. These are hugely significant developments."

Despite changing demographics, elders have always yearned for independence and control, said Andrew Achenbaum, professor of history and social work at University of Houston. Society as a whole has voiced ambivalence about the meaning of old age. In his book, *Old Age in the New Land*, Achenbaum wrote, "Philosophers, poets and other writers for millennia have pondered the aged's strengths and weaknesses and alternately affirmed the potential and despaired the decline that comes with age."[2]

On one hand, older people were seen as wise counselors with a highly developed sense of morality. The loss and frailty that accompanies old age were understood to give elders more compassion and wisdom than younger people who had not yet faced life's trials, and older people were viewed with respect and admiration. This view was most commonly held in the United States before the Civil War, according to Achenbaum's research, when retirement was not mandatory and people worked as long as they were able.

But the view of old people as somehow different from the rest of the population was a mixed blessing. Eventually their status was undermined, and the shift to labeling old people as "the other" began. "Instead of depicting the elderly as stately and healthy, more and more observers described them as ugly and disease-ridden," Achenbaum wrote of the post-Civil War era.

By the twentieth century old people were seen as a vexing problem. They were portrayed as physically and cognitively in decline, economically useless in the industrial age, sometimes even deviant in their behavior. Moreover, the popular press focused on all manner of disagreeable qualities supposedly common in the elderly; they were presented as being bitter, grumpy, lazy, judgmental, unkempt.

Once they became viewed as a problem, then of course they needed to be "fixed." Eventually a vast network of solutions to the "problem" of old age was developed, including the development of tens of thousands of nursing homes, assisted living and retirement communities, and now a $100 billion industry in "anti-aging" products. Increasingly, younger to middle-aged adults came to be viewed as "normal," and older people as "less than." A 2013 study led by Becca Levy of the Yale School of Public Health documented extreme ageism on Facebook, the popular social media site, identifying eighty-four groups (made up of more than 25,000 members) that, according to their own descriptions, focused on older people. Of these groups, all but one were sites where people espoused extremely negative views, with one group even proclaiming that anyone "over the age of 69 should immediately face a firing squad," while other groups described elders as "infantile" people who should not be allowed to drive or shop.[3]

Increasingly, though, researchers, advocates, and older people themselves have pushed back against long-held ageism. In an article on aging in place, scholars writing about "naturally occurring retirement communities" (NORCs; see Chapter 6) challenged the assumption that being old, by definition, means being frail, vulnerable, and helpless. They suggest that powerful images and stereotypes have the force of self-fulfilling prophecy. They point to a body of research that has found that older people who believe they have something valuable to contribute to their families and their communities and who assume they will not end up in institutions actually feel healthier and are much more likely to successfully age in place than their peers who hold more negative views about their lives. The researchers called for fundamentally changing our "images and perceptions of needy, dependent older adults," replacing them with "images and perceptions of older adults as wise, resilient, and capable of offering resources to their communities." This transformation, the researchers suggest, actually promotes our ability to age in place.[4]

This goes along with what the SCAN Foundation and other researchers have found. "At some level all of us really want to be the person we are today and we don't want to see ourselves as functionally limited tomorrow," said Bruce Chernof. "Most people want to see themselves as good and hard-working and successful."

☙☙

Dale, a striking eighty-year-old widow who lives in a lake community outside Columbia, South Carolina, reflected on her conflicted feelings about this time of life. "It's hard to believe I'm actually eighty," she said with a laugh. "The only reason I wouldn't care for someone to know how old I am is we have so many stereotypes. I hate the thought of being stereotyped—the 'daftness' [people associate with old age]."

Dale, who still drives at night, lives alone, has a full life with friends and family, and is a youthful-looking and beautiful woman, does not fit the image that most people probably carry in their heads of octogenarians. I met her at a friends' gathering on a boat dock, where we drank wine and watched July fourth fireworks over Lake Murray. In this and later conversations, what struck me about Dale was her thoughtful consideration of what her future might hold.

As Dale illustrates, the definition of "old" grows ever more malleable. Does getting a Social Security check and receiving Medicare in your mid-sixties make you "old"? After all, when the Social Security Act was passed in 1935 one of the main purposes was to ensure that older Americans did not live in desperate poverty. It was called "old-age assistance." But I venture to guess that few of the baby boomers getting ready to collect their "old age assistance" feel *old*. Now we have terms like "old-old" for people over eighty-five, and even that is not always descriptive. The very notion of chronological age is being questioned: a sixty-five-year old with multiple chronic medical conditions and poor mobility may share much with a ninety-year old in a nursing home, while someone like Dale may be much "younger" than her age would suggest.

In a *New York Times* "New Old Age" blog, experts were asked what to call this demographic group now that baby boomers are among its youngest members.[5] There was little agreement—seniors, elders, the elderly—none seemed quite right. Even the word "aging" itself is so associated with decline that many reject it. (Teddi, seventy-six and a resident of the Burbank Senior Artists Colony, told me she preferred the term "recycled teen.")

"The culture's problem is that we split aging into good and bad," Thomas Cole, director of the McGovern Center for Humanities and Ethics at the University of Texas Health Science Center at Houston, wrote on the blog. "We're unable to sustain images of growing older that handle the tension between spiritual growth, the good, and physical decline, the bad. In the Hebrew Bible, aging is both a blessing and a curse. But our culture can't achieve this kind of synthesis."

A senior cohousing community in Santa Fe even decided to change its name from ElderGrace to Sand River because of the connotation. "The main reason is, we have some men in our community who didn't want to tell anybody where they lived—they felt it created an image of gray-haired people walking around with walkers," explained Marty, a resident there. "People asked if it was assisted living. I actually had someone I ran into who came to dinner and she asked if we'd sold the last two units in 'ElderCare.' That convinced me."

In a 2013 piece on NPR headlined "For Elderly Midwife, Delivering Babies Never Gets Old," about a seventy-one-year-old practitioner, a huge outcry erupted over the label "elderly," including a complaint from the midwife.[6] (As an example of how language evolves, one commenter on a *Washington Post* blog reminded readers that humorist Stan Freeburg in 1957 rewrote the lyrics to a classic show tune, singing "Elderly Man River," since the word "old" had been censored.[7]) In fact, journalists are now advised to avoid any descriptor such as "elderly" for fear of offending someone. "Use this word carefully and sparingly," according to the *Associated Press Stylebook*.[8]

Many writers have tried to make sense of this new era. "Anti-aging" books have been published for the last twenty years, promising elixirs that will keep our bodies youthful, our sex drive in fourth gear, our skin petal-fresh, and our lifespan stretched well past the century mark. Others reject these promises as naive at best, hucksterism at worst. Instead, some argue, we need to embrace our Inner Elder, reclaiming our rightful place as wisdom-holders and keepers of the flame. Some see the Third Age—the stage between the Second Age of employment and childrearing and the Fourth Age during our last chapter of life—as a time of liberation, forever young on our own terms, with retirement as rediscovery.

Although most would welcome this, the truth is that old age is a frontier that none of us can predict until we're trekking through the middle of it. How our health—physical, emotional, cognitive—holds up depends on our genes, our environment, and our lifestyle, and to pretend otherwise can leave us unprepared to face serious difficulties that are bound to arise. Millions of us face financial hardship as well, challenging our expectations of what old age will be like.

We would do well to contemplate the next chapter of our lives. What will our homes be like? If, like my mother, we begin to fall or have difficulty walking or our vision fails, will our home serve us or be an impediment to our wellbeing? How will the fabric of our lives be woven? Are there people nearby—family, neighbors, friends, members of our congregation—who care about us, who would be willing to help us or accept help from us?

The essential question facing each of us as we age is: how can we balance our desire for independence with staying connected to others? That we even can raise this question is remarkable. Never before have older people, often through their own imagination and determination, had real options from which to choose.

ℭℨℭ

In modern US culture, the concept of "retirement living" was born in 1955, in Youngtown, Arizona, the nation's first age-segregated retirement community. This was followed in 1960 by Sun City, the brainchild of developer Del Webb. According to the corporate website: "Spurred on by the early success of Youngtown . . . Webb Company officials developed the idea of taking the 'retirement' community concept to the next level. Youngtown was created for retirees living on minimal, fixed incomes. The homes were small—the amenities nonexistent. Del Webb toyed with the idea of creating a self-sustaining community that would be all encompassing with affordable housing and recreation."[9] In 1962, Del Webb made the cover of *Time* magazine, with the headline, "A new way of life for the old."[10] (Never mind that in the accompanying story we learn that the hard-charging Webb "could not stand the life in one of his own Sun Cities for more than a few days—or a few hours.")

Today there are fifty-nine Del Webb communities, forty-four of them age-restricted, with golf courses, swimming pools, wellness centers, lifelong learning opportunities, art studios, and clubs. According to the website, "everyone plays a part, everyone brings something to the party. So chart a new course, start fresh, free your inhibitions, let yourself shine at Del Webb."

Much as the "active seniors" want to believe they will be lobbing tennis balls until the end, frailty and forgetfulness sneak up. This was recognized by the next iteration of elder housing which came in the 1970s with assisted living, essentially the "NOT-nursing home" alternative for those who could no longer live independently. Assisted living encompasses a spectrum, from very modest single rooms to full, accessible apartments (often minus the stove, for safety reasons). Residents are provided meals and assistance as needed. In nearly 90 percent of cases, people pay for assisted living out of pocket. Although nominally considered "independent" living, assisted living increasingly attracts people with dementia and chronic medical conditions.

From there emerged "continuing care retirement communities," offering a spectrum of living options, as people's health declines and they need more services. These communities claim to give people the chance to age in place. But in many, if not most, of these communities, independent residents must move to a different building on the campus for assisted living, and then again for the nursing home, making "aging in place" somewhat illusory. There is often considerable stigma toward those who need more services, and friendships forged as independent residents may fray with each move toward needing more help.

Then of course there is the nursing home, where so many grandparents spend their final weeks, months, or years. Truly the last resort, nursing homes have been slow to catch on to how deeply flawed and soul-killing an institutional culture can be for anyone, including vulnerable older people. For nearly twenty years, the "culture change" movement has sought to transform nursing homes from hospital-like facilities, with shared bedrooms, rigid mealtimes, prescribed activities, and top-down rules, to warm, caring communities where people feel at least some sense of friendship and "home." But change is excruciatingly slow, and despite wonderful models that demonstrate a high quality of life is possible, it's safe to say almost everyone fears having a nursing home in their future.

Will my generation do things differently? That's the question that today's developers of retirement communities (also called "amenitized" or "active adult" communities in the trade) are eager to figure out. But pinning down an entire generation—the largest one at that—is a tricky business. Marketing publications aimed at developers breezily describe my generation as if we had all gone to Woodstock. As one advises: "Know Your Market. Baby Boomers are not like their parents. They dedicated their younger years to rebelling against their parents and their lifestyles. You also need to recognize that the leading edge Baby Boomers who led the social revolutions of the 1960s are different from the younger Baby Boomers who brought us the 'Me Decade' of the 1970s." (Whatever that bit of insight means.) The same article proclaims that for boomers "the environment is king," and "the original flower children loved nature and always will." Luckily, it continues, "the environment is the cheapest thing you can add to your development; think hiking trails, nature preserves, community gardens."[11]

(Interestingly, according to a Del Webb survey these graying rebels tend to describe themselves as "conservative;" their top three heroes are not Bob Dylan, Martin Luther King, or John F. Kennedy, but "Mom, Dad, family; Jesus, God; and Ronald Reagan," in that order.)[12]

The sheer volume of aging Americans gives developers reason to be giddy. According to an upbeat 2013 market analysis, nearly fifteen thousand retirement community businesses earn a combined $54 billion in annual revenue, and those numbers are growing more than 3 percent a year.[13]

But despite that heady optimism, and no matter how many yoga classes, hiking trails, and gourmet kitchens developers offer, it may be a tough sell. The truth is only a fraction of people are attracted to—or can afford—retirement communities as we know them.

According to data by the National Association of Homebuilders, 63 percent of us plan to stay put, 12 percent hope to buy a different home, and 26 percent are undecided. The Del Webb survey of baby boomers found that 32 percent of older "leading-edge" boomers, already sixty-four years old, planned to move, and 42 percent of younger boomers planned to relocate in retirement. Of those planning to move, though, only a small portion expressed a preference for an age-restricted retirement community.[14] A Metlife Mature Market Institute report found that just over one million of the nearly forty million people aged fifty-five and older own a home in an age-restricted (the industry prefers the more sunny term, "age-qualified") community, with another 1.5 million renting.[15]

Carol, eighty-four, visited traditional retirement communities before moving to ElderSpirit, a cohousing community in Virginia. "I call them luxury warehousing," she said. "I couldn't stand it. You don't see a lot of active people. It's soul-eroding."

Many others have critiqued retirement communities. Maggie Kuhn, founder of the Gray Panthers, dubbed them "glorified playpens for seniors" and physician and author Muriel Gillick described them as "sterile, artificial."[16] In his scathing book *Leisureville: Adventures in a World Without Children* writer Andrew M. Blechman documented a culture where elders devote day after day to an endless round of games and cocktail parties, living in a closed environment where occupants have turned their backs on the world at large.[17]

This is not to say that retirement communities do not offer their occupants a good life. Many do. My friend Norma, a close confidant of my mother's, has lived in a Methodist continuing care retirement community for decades, the same one where my mother moved. Norma assures me that they have true community there and that many of the outstanding educational and cultural offerings they have were initiated by residents themselves. Living among her peers—the highly educated and affluent elders here in Montgomery County, Maryland—she is contented. There are many such communities.

Others are hardly luxurious, but have been seen by northern retirees as a well-earned and affordable reward in a sunny Southern climate. The reality, though, does not always meet their expectations. In the 2012 documentary of her grandmother's retirement community in Florida, *Kings Point*, where residents are far older than what you see in a Del Webb ad, filmmaker Sari Gilman captured an atmosphere of loneliness and quiet desperation amid the card games and tap dancing at the Monaco Clubhouse. "You try to fill the days as best you can—you go to the mall, movies on Friday, play mahjong. In other words you make the best of living in Florida," said one resident. "No one gets close here—they're afraid. Everybody is a user here," offered another. And perhaps most poignant: "When you were younger you made friend-friends. When you came to Florida you made acquaintances—and good acquaintances. Not friend-friends. They're just not here anymore."

It's hard to imagine most of my friends and acquaintances choosing such a life, although a fraction of my generation will. According to market surveys, those who are uprooting often do move for the climate, just as their parents did, although the Carolinas have edged out Florida as the top destination.

Another small group will reject settling down at all, at least while they are healthy and fit enough to travel. A recent Reuters story reported on "rambling retirees" who sell their homes and live on houseboats, in recreational vehicles (RVs), or even crash on sofas and in guest rooms through an online network of hospitality. Although firm statistics are scarce, some nine thousand retirees reportedly live on the water and twenty-five thousand in RVs.[18]

Other observers say the baby boomers will indeed demand something different from the traditional retirement community. At a seminar I attended at Harvard in 2008, Maria Dwight, president of the consulting firm Gerontological Services, Inc., noted that "Not only are most of the physical plants of yesteryear outdated and unattractive to the market—the rules, regulations, and routines are passé as well." She predicted that communities that are "traditional management-centric" would lose out to those that are "resident centric."

Indeed, even the nicest retirement communities often have rules that many of us would chafe under, such as not allowing candles (due to fire concerns), banning pets, and restricting the length of time that grandchildren can visit.

A 2012 report by the Urban Land Institute, "Housing in America: The Baby Boomers Turn 65," found that older people now represent three distinct "market segments"—the Greatest Generation, the Silent Generation, and baby boomers—each with different outlooks and needs. While noting the recurring theme that most people want to remain in their own homes, many who choose to move are gravitating toward places with vibrant "town centers," near their grown children, friends, work, public transportation, and health care. "Leading-edge boomers will not settle gracefully into quiet retirement and move into traditional seniors housing communities for years, if they ever do," writes ULI Senior Resident Fellow for Housing John K. McIlwain. Other studies reach a similar conclusion.

That may be closer to the mark. But how different is my generation? The ULI report goes on to note that the baby boomers "are not alone in their antipathy to institutional living," and that "they share this sentiment with their parents." As Nat Yalowitz, eighty-four, a leader of Penn South Cooperative in Manhattan wrote: "[Seniors] don't want to be 'entertained' according to someone else's view of what they need. They want to have a major say as to what types of programs will best serve their needs. They resist any ageism on the part of staff in various institutions they go to."[19]

Perhaps we're not so terribly unique in what we want. What may be different, though, is our confidence and willingness to take risks and to create communities that please us. Many in my generation have two strong streaks that may serve us well as we grow old. One is a desire for agency and control and a resistance to passivity and authority for authority's sake that exhibited itself in both the political and the personal. The other is a recognition of the importance of community and a willingness to invest ourselves in long-lasting relationships.

For some of us, the desire to resist authority meant organizing mass movements to protest the Vietnam War, demand civil rights, and advocate for women's equality. On a personal level, it led us to transform the experience of childbirth from a medicalized procedure in which women were "knocked out" in an operating room where the doctors proceeded to deliver a baby to one where women and their partners are the main actors in the drama, receiving training through childbirth classes and going through labor and delivery in homey settings where they are coached by nurse midwives and doulas. Mothers of my generation also began to return to nursing their babies, rather than feeding them industrial formula in a bottle.

At the same time, the so-called Me Generation has had a healthy regard for communitarianism and for changing their local communities and the world. Families organized babysitting co-ops or cooperative nurseries. We created community gardens and local farmers markets; organized fundraising walks for all manner of charities; led the effort to make recycling an expected duty of municipalities; and so on. We were instrumental (although hardly alone) in what activist and author Paul Hawken—himself a leading-edge baby boomer—calls "Blessed Unrest," a global outpouring of an estimated one million local organizations working on environmentalism and social justice.[20]

These two seemingly contradictory traits—autonomy and community— are precisely what can transform the experience of millions of older people. They no longer see life in "solitary confinement" in their own homes or in top-down retirement communities and long-term care institutions that are so distasteful to so many as their only choices.

"There are a lot of us baby boomers who have seen our parents struggle with a broken system," said Robert Jenkens, senior vice president and director of social impact initiatives of the National Cooperative Bank and a long-time supporter of transformative eldercare. "Baby boomers are old enough to say something has to change so this will be acceptable for our parents and for us. There's a lot of energy around this, and a lot of creativity and capacity and people with more money to do this."

A few years ago, I got wind of alternative ways to live that appealed to me; ways that I could imagine for my husband and me, my sister, and friends. People were spending energy, time, resources, and creativity to reimagine their lives after—or even before—retirement.

One model that has received considerable press attention is called the Village, a neighbors-helping-neighbors membership organization that is popping up around the country. "I'm so convinced that these Villages are part of a major cultural shift in our society," said Sonia Crow, former director of Palisades Village in Washington, DC. "There's some terrible loss that's happened to us culturally. People feel such gaps in their sense of community, of caring, of connection."

Ann Zabaldo, who lives in a cohousing community in Washington, DC, agrees. "On a deeper level," she said, "across the board there's a yearning for connectedness."

The same could be said of all the alternatives ways of living in this book: each is an effort by people not only to remain independent throughout their lives but, as importantly, to have connections to others. Indeed, aging advocate Steve Gurney, publisher of a retirement resource book in the Washington, DC, area, suggested to me that the notion of "independence" should be abolished in favor of "interdependence."

This book has at its heart the stories of individuals who recognize the value of interdependence, who refuse to accept the status quo, who dare to imagine a life different from that of their parents in old age and then dedicate themselves to making that vision a reality. In this way, the alternatives here are different from a traditional developer-built retirement community. For some, like those in Villages or NORCs (naturally occurring retirement communities), this means joining forces with others in their communities to organize ways for neighbors to help each other. For some it is the ambitious undertaking of constructing a whole new intentional cohousing community that is comprised either of older people or of multiple generations. Others share a house with close friends—or even strangers—to have an affordable lifestyle with steadfast companionship. Or they create living situations with an affinity group, whether based on sexual orientation, religion, the arts, or other common interest. Still others establish cooperatives of manufactured housing in rural areas or apartments in urban centers. And others live with extended family, but in ways perhaps more reciprocal and interdependent than in the past. Some options, such as many cohousing communities, may require substantial financial resources, usually available to those who bought homes as young adults and are able to sell them decades later for a hefty profit. But I also searched for affordable options and I found many. The blossoming of possibilities continues, even as I write this, with some yet to be imagined.

CHAPTER 2

Interdependence

Reconsidering "Aging in Place"

The flowering of alternative ways to live grows out of the desire to "age in place." For years, aging in place has been the mantra of AARP and many specialists in aging. It's no surprise. Survey after survey shows that the vast majority of older people say that is their wish and their plan.

Dale, who lives on Lake Murray in South Carolina, explained why aging in place is so appealing to her. As we grow older, she said, "the familiar" takes on growing importance. "Just being every day around the things that have become such a part of your life," she says of why she treasures remaining in her own home. "It might be a little risky sometimes as people get a bit physically unstable or whatever, but if you're in your own home you still know how to get around, you know where things are. It's just so delightful, for me, to think of being surrounded by my own home rather than picked up and moved to some strange place, even though you might have help there."

On a deeper level, she said, staying in her home of many years gives her a sense of identity and history that would be threatened by uprooting. Of her grandchildren's recent summer visit, she said, "It was just wonderful. I wanted them to know me in my home and where I have activities and a boat and they can catch frogs outside and swim in the lake and see it as a home—not some institution that they visit."

Moreover, she has a strong sense of community right where she is. "I don't enjoy just being with women or with people the same age," she said. "I love being able to interact with couples and people of all different age groups. It's hard to make a move to even a retirement village as a single eighty-year-old, to make new friends. . . . When you go somewhere brand new, you have no history. They didn't know your husband and the humor that he had and what a good preacher he was and your children. It's as though you've lost your past a little bit."

Of course not everyone has what Dale has. Aging in place is only as good as the place you're aging in. Nat Yalowitz, a long-time leader of Penn South Cooperative, noted, "When we promote the home as the place where we hope and expect the senior might 'age in place,' we put a great deal of faith in the senior's home being a positive influence in the senior's life. We don't necessarily bother to examine the home situation and the senior living there from a dynamic point of view."[1]

"Home" can be especially challenging for those living in poverty. As researcher Stephen Golant of the University of Florida observed, "Most experts, professionals, and practitioners, along with older persons themselves, have elevated the aging in place response to the status of an indisputable truth." Golant "questions this unbridled enthusiasm," arguing that "staying put is sometimes an inappropriate strategy to address the housing and care needs of lower-income older homeowners. A better alternative is for these persons to seek out different housing arrangements that are more congruent with their late life health declines and financial constraints."[2]

It's not only lower-income people who may find aging in place has its challenges. Many older people, regardless of financial status, are "over-housed," meaning their homes are much larger than they need. Aging at home can mean clinging to a home they can no longer afford or maintain. A 2010 MetLife study examined the complex array of support services and technology that needs to be developed for aging in place to succeed. "Though almost everyone says they want to Age in Place, individuals or families trying to assist an older relative may find it difficult. Organizing, confirming, and managing care and services can be a daunting task because the delivery system is often fragmented, and needed services may be difficult to find or not always available in an individual's local area."[3]

Of practical concern, most houses were not constructed with the idea that occupants may lose mobility. Stairs can be an enormous obstacle. My mother moved to a retirement community after one fall too many—the last one as she carried a basket of clean clothes up from the laundry room in the split-level house where she'd lived for forty-five years, resulting in two broken wrists. The house couldn't have been built in a worse way for growing old in: to access a bathroom or bedroom required going up and down stairs, and there was no space on the main floor to adapt or add on.

Stairs are only one of many potential obstacles in our homes; there are also light switches that you can't reach if you're in a wheelchair, fixtures and knobs difficult to operate with arthritic hands, cabinets so high you must climb on a footstool to access them, and so on (see Chapter 12).

Even something as simple as dragging your garbage cans to the curb can become daunting, if not impossible. When she reached that point, my late neighbor, June, began looking at retirement communities. Even though we and other neighbors assured her we'd be happy to carry out that task for her, she hated to impose.

Then there's transportation. If you live in the suburbs or a rural area, driving is practically mandatory unless you are willing to face great limits on your ability to get out of your house. Even if you have the means to pay for taxis, they are often unreliable or unavailable, as is public transit. My then-ninety-four-year-old mother-in-law, determined to remain independent, took a cab to a shopping mall and got stranded when she wanted to return home. When she called for a cab, it never came. With her usual resourcefulness and chutzpah, she approached a couple and asked them for a ride, which they graciously gave her. ("He was wearing a yarmulke," she explained later, which apparently made the total stranger seem like a safe bet.)

In southern Montgomery County, Maryland, where I live, an interfaith group of volunteers, many of them older themselves, helps people get to medical appointments and the grocery—a welcome and important contribution, but life is about more than medical appointments. Going to a movie or a museum, shopping, or visiting friends can be extremely challenging, especially after dark, and without convenient transportation frail older people become increasingly isolated.

And that leads to perhaps the biggest potential problem with aging, whether "in place" or in some sort of group or institutional setting: loneliness, boredom, and helplessness. In an August 2012 blog posting, geriatrician Bill Thomas, founder of the Eden Alternative and Green House approaches to eldercare, wrote, "The myth of 'aging in place' harms people by defining the decision to share one's daily life with others as failure. But a big piece of the reluctance to seek out new ways of living with others is the dread of institutionalization. People cling to their homes in large part because they fear life in a nursing home more than they fear death."[4]

Oz Ragland, an advocate for both cohousing and housesharing who lives near Seattle, gave the example of his father-in-law whom he said is in "an archetypal bad situation." At eighty-six, his father-in-law lives alone and is beginning to have serious memory problems. "The family is clustered around trying to figure out what to do with this guy," said Oz. "He has no support network whatsoever, other than his family. He has six kids, but they're spread all over the world."

The desire to stay autonomous and live by your own rules can come at a steep price. A public health physician in Great Britain wrote an essay lamenting this isolation. Over the Christmas holidays she visited one of her depressed older patients who lived alone and later wrote "It brings home to me the truth of this epidemic that we have on our hands—an epidemic of loneliness, insidiously affecting those among us who have seen the ebb and flow of countless seasons."[5]

Many who cling to aging in place awake one day to realize just how lonely that place has become. In fact, rescue squads often field calls from lonely older people who long for a human connection. In Upper Arlington, a suburb of Columbus, Ohio, for example, the fire and police departments complain of receiving 911 calls from older people not because of any emergencies but because they want companionship or help with a simple household task. Police call these "lonely complainant 911 calls."[6] Researchers who are examining the use of technologies like lifeline pendants by older adults report a similar phenomenon. (See Chapter 15.)

The strong desire to age in place, even in the face of loneliness, is not inherent, but rather stems from our culture's fierce defense of autonomy. According to scholars, beginning in 1950 there was a significant shift in the number of older people living alone. Researchers have different theories about the cause. For one, rising incomes allowed them to, perhaps for the first time. In other words, older people may have always wanted more independence but could not afford it in the past. In addition, with smaller families, fewer adult children were able or willing to take them in. Traditional family values also were in flux. "Personal preferences for privacy and independence may, in part, be the result of societal norms," according to researchers. "Thus, the extent to which elders perceive a social expectation that they *should* manage on their own until physically unable may contribute to some of their stated desire for private and independent styles of living."[7]

Advocates for cohousing maintain that living in community trumps any perceived benefit that comes from living alone. "Aging in place is pandering to old people because that's what they want to hear," insisted Ann Zabaldo, a leader in the cohousing movement. "So they come up with 'smart houses' [which have technology installed to be able to monitor old people]. The only thing you've done is isolate people more and more, instead of educating people about the importance of interconnectedness. That's what keeps you young—it's your relatedness, it's being involved in your life."

Ann added that it's unsustainable and unrealistic to think that seventy-two million baby boomers can continue to live in their own homes as they become frail and need more support. Her views are supported by study after study suggesting that loneliness undermines our health and well-being and, conversely, that close companionship has important benefits.

Friends and family are essential to a full, happy, and purposeful life. Two-thirds of people age forty-five and over said being near friends and/or family was extremely or very important, according to an AARP survey.[8] Although this may sound too obvious to mention (wouldn't people of any age say this?), we often seem to accept without question older people's lack of regular companionship. We may not fully appreciate the toll that loneliness can take. Researchers have found real risks to our health from social isolation and loneliness, which negatively influences stress hormones, immune system functioning, blood pressure, and levels of inflammation, making us vulnerable to an array of illnesses and conditions.

Researchers in Great Britain followed 6,500 people aged fifty-two and older who participated in the English Longitudinal Study of Aging in 2004–2005. The researchers examined, among other things, participants' loneliness and social isolation and then in 2012 looked at mortality statistics for the group. Social isolation was judged in terms of contact with family and friends or involvement in civic organizations. They found that social isolation contributed to dying; 21.9 percent of those in the "high isolation" group had died, compared to 12.3 percent in the "low isolation" group, after controlling for other factors. They cited troubling statistics about the trend toward social isolation:

> Social isolation is a growing problem among middle-aged and older people. In 2011, people living alone comprised 28% of all households in the United States, compared with 17% in 1970. The proportion of Americans who said they had no one to talk to about important matters increased from 10% in 1985 to 25% in 2004. . . . Between 1996 and 2012, the proportion of people aged 45–64 who lived alone in England and Wales rose by 53%.[9]

In contrast, a 2010 study of 279 British retirees found that being involved in social networks was strongly correlated with life satisfaction—surprisingly, more so than having children or grandchildren. "These findings support the importance of interventions designed to promote social networking in those who could experience retirement as a lonely, rather than fulfilling, stage of life," noted the researcher, Dr. Oliver Robinson of University of Greenwich.[10]

My seventy-something-year-old friend Marty told me of her play-reading group that has been meeting for forty-seven years. As group members grew older, the act of reading a script became difficult for some. One now has Alzheimer's, and while he still can read, he has difficulty focusing. Another had a stroke and while he is on the road to rehabilitation, he cannot read. Rather than continue without them or disband, the group is trying different formats. First they tried attending plays, but they couldn't agree on which to go to. Now they're going to try eating out together—if they can find a restaurant quiet enough for those with hearing loss. Marty (who is hard of hearing) laughed as she told me this. "We are so determined not to give up," she said.

That's what we should all be working toward, it seems to me: having a group around us who won't give up on us, who wants to hang out with us through thick and thin, who won't let us be pushed aside. It doesn't really matter whether you find that in your hometown neighborhood or cooperative, in a new intentional community, or in sharing a house with friends. The secret to a high quality of life as we grow old is being known and appreciated for who we are—and to offer that friendship to others.

That doesn't mean that people who live alone are doomed to unhappiness—which may come as welcome news to single people tired of hearing about a correlation between longevity and marriage. What may be harmful, though, to our sense of well-being is not having confidants or companions.[11]

A study published in 2011 suggests a health advantage of living in a close-knit community.[12] Researchers developed a "cohesion" scale for neighborhoods. People were asked if they spoke with their neighbors in the street, did yard work together, took care of neighborhood children, or otherwise looked out for one another. They found that among 5,789 older men and women in Chicago, the higher the cohesion, the higher the chance of survival following a stroke. (For reasons not determined, the same survival benefit did not apply in African American neighborhoods that had high cohesion.)

Having a network of friends was associated with ten-year survival in a longitudinal study of 1,177 people aged seventy and older in Australia. At the end of ten years, after controlling for health and other variables, the researchers found that the 570 people who were still alive had larger networks of friends than their counterparts who had died. Interestingly, the same protective effect was not found for those whose social network was made up of relatives. The researchers speculated: "Friends possibly also encourage health seeking behaviour, which in turn can affect survival. Friends can have effects on depression, self efficacy, self esteem, coping and morale, or a sense of personal control, possibly through social engagement by reinforcing social roles or because interactions with friends stem from choice or selectivity."[13]

A longitudinal study called Midlife in the United States (MIDUS) has followed a group of seven thousand people since 1994. One part of the study asked people if they felt younger or older than their chronological age. Those who felt younger were not only healthier, as we would expect, but they also felt they had more control over their lives and a greater sense of purpose. They were more likely to volunteer, to spend time with friends, and to regularly attend religious services. "Adults who feel younger are also more likely to feel that they have contributed positively to others over the course of their lives, with 70% reporting contributions to others that have been excellent or very good in comparison to 54% of adults who feel older," the study found.[14]

Although feeling younger than one's age is not necessarily a goal in itself, what it connotes is certainly more positive than feeling older than one's age. Presumably those who feel younger than their age are relatively healthy, feel optimistic about the future, and have a reason to get out of bed in the morning.

Other researchers look at the oldest-old and what contributes to healthy longevity. In his book *The Blue Zones*, on communities around the globe with an unusually high portion of centenarians, science writer Dan Buettner identified nine common behaviors that may help us live long and well.[15]

- Incorporate movement into your everyday routine
- Eat about 80 percent of your normal diet
- Limit meat and processed foods
- Regularly have a drink or two of wine or beer
- Have a sense of purpose
- Make time for relaxation and socialization
- Be part of a spiritual community
- Make family a priority
- Surround yourself with others who share these behaviors

Research such as this bolsters the hope that "aging in community"—more than "aging in place"—may act as a buffer to protect us from problems associated with growing old. In fact, aging in place at all costs can backfire. In his book *Senior Cohousing*, Charles Durrett bemoans that despite his best efforts to convince his mother to move to cohousing, she chose the path that so many older people do: aging in place, which can also look a lot like living in denial. "She was determined to live out her days on her 'own terms,'" he writes, "telling herself that she was in complete control. Nobody was going to tell her what to do and how to live."[16]

Ten years later, she spent her last chapter in an institutional nursing home where "she has no choice but to live according to the whims and timetables set by the staff . . . she lives alone among strangers, her chance to make a deliberate and realistic choice as to how and where she would live out her last years long since past."[17]

Whether choosing to live more intentionally as part of a community, however you define that, will protect us from ending our days in a nursing home is too soon to tell. The movement to reinvent our Third Age is in its infancy and many questions remain. Will basing our older years on "interdependence" delay or even preclude the need for costly, dreaded, institutional long-term care, as some advocates maintain? Will focusing on both autonomy and social connectedness help people stay healthier? What about Alzheimer's and other diseases that cause dementia—can these conditions be delayed, or, if not, well-managed in a caring community?

For some, personal choices about living arrangements involve broader issues beyond one's own aging. How do we live simply and sustainably, conserving Earth's resources? What about those on fixed incomes—are there appealing options that are affordable and accessible to people in poorer communities? How well integrated into the full life of a community, with people of all ages, are elders, and does this matter?

As discussed, we baby boomers are famous for reinventing ourselves and society. If my generation can proactively take on the challenge of growing old with grace, humor, and intention, that would be progress indeed. My wish is that instead of pretending we will live forever young, until a crisis forces us to realize we're not, we will ponder the big questions: Which of the many ways to live will I choose? What will give my life the most meaning and joy? How will I get myself from here to there?

Denial, long the drink of choice for those facing their twilight happy hours, no longer seems so appealing to many of my peers. And that is a welcome development. Because only by facing this stage of life, by really thinking about what is possible—and what is not—can we do what all of us want: to maintain our independence, a sense of autonomy, and the connections that give our lives purpose and happiness.

PART II

A Wealth of Options

CHAPTER 3

The Village
Neighbors Helping Neighbors

In the English basement of a townhouse in Washington, DC, the first call of the day came into Capitol Hill Village. Pauline, a member, said she needed potatoes, Dawn dish detergent, and the chicken that was on sale at Harris Teeter supermarket.

No problem. Patrick, a volunteer, would take care of it.

Next up: a member needed a house sitter for two days. She had to be away from home, and she wanted someone to wait for a repairman. Gail Kohn, who at that time was the organization's director, opened the computer file of members and scanned through the list. She paused and looked over her glasses at Lois, the volunteer receptionist that day. "You know, Lois, I'm looking for feelings of self-worth," she observed. "I'm not looking at ways to make it easy."

Lois nodded.

Translation: at Capitol Hill Village, the goal is for each member of the organization to have opportunities to contribute to the common good. In this case, a man willing to house sit had difficulty walking and needed transportation to get there—requiring yet another volunteer. But that was okay.

"Two-thirds of our work is creating community, not providing services," Gail explained. Gail has worked in the field of eldercare for decades. When she heard of the Village concept—an organized way that neighbors could help each other remain in their own homes—she was sold.

Of the many new ways to age in community people are creating, the fastest growing may be the Village model. Initiated in the Beacon Hill neighborhood of Boston in 2002, Villages generally rely on a mix of paid staff and volunteers to assist older residents with everything from transportation to computer know-how, dog walking, and grocery shopping. Members pay annual dues and are encouraged to volunteer themselves. Villages also organize social events, exercise classes, personal finance workshops—whatever members want.

"When we started, we were having lectures and seminars," said Sonia Crow, the former executive director of Palisades Village, also in Washington, DC. "But we learned people weren't terribly interested in things like reverse mortgages. We learned from our members what they'd really like is to sit down and talk with someone, maybe have something nice to eat or drink. These Villages force you to pause and actually listen and be responsive to what people want."

Capitol Hill Village, with 360 members living in 265 households, is one of the nation's largest. The organization benefits not only from Gail Kohn's leadership and fundraising acumen but also from free office space. The English basement is cream-painted brick, long and narrow, with a conference table surrounded by desks in the front room. The owner, who lives in the townhouse above, travels frequently and was happy to have the organization set up shop below. He even lets them spill over to the upstairs when more privacy is needed, such as when the social worker on staff—the only paid employee other than Gail—needs to consult with a member. Behind the main room is a full kitchen, with bottles of wine and cans of cashews—the latter, Gail's main sustenance—on the counter.

On a warm September day, the phone rang steadily. While Gail was on one line, another call came in from someone needing a ride downtown. Gail immediately returned the call. "I don't know who will take you, but one of us will," she said. She listened to the response. "I'm not questioning why you're getting your calculator repaired. If Al will repair it for you, cool."

She hung up. In fact, she did wonder if a fifteen-year-old calculator was worth repairing, but if the member was sure that a particular employee at a particular bookshop would fix it, who was she to question?

"It takes someone like Gail to make this work," Patrick, the volunteer, commented. He doesn't live on Capitol Hill, but enjoyed helping out. He offered an example of how Gail's vision comes to life. "There's a guy in Silver Spring [a Maryland suburb] whose mother lives on Capitol Hill. He came and cooked for her and laid out her medications. But he wanted help from Capitol Hill Village to check on her. Gail realized there was another member on the same block. She connected the two. Now they look out for each other and share meals sometimes. So rather than having someone checking in on her in a patronizing way, she's in mutual support with a member," he said. "I tend to think mechanistically. Gail doesn't."

Or take the member who had a knee replacement. He could have been purely a recipient of help, asking for grocery delivery or housekeeping. But in an organizational culture that stresses reciprocity and interdependence, he wanted to do his part. He ended up playing an important role for Capitol Hill Village, making calls from his home to see if members were satisfied with the volunteer help they'd received. The organization has a strong system of accountability, with every member who receives a service asked to evaluate how it went.

The week before, someone had donated a Singer sewing machine to the organization. It's now on loan to a member. "She doesn't want someone to sew for her," said Gail. "She wants to do it herself."

Judy, another volunteer, arrived at the office. "I think of the Village as a grassroots movement that's popping up all over the place," she said. Judy is a charter member and volunteer. A few years ago, she was having medical issues and was constantly going to the doctor. "I learned how important it was to have support," she said. "Friends and neighbors were helping me with transportation and meals." When a friend told her about Capitol Hill Village, she decided to join, even though it was a leap of faith. "I thought of it as an investment," she said.

One benefit she enjoys is having a "rise and shine partner," designed for members who live alone. The two speak every morning and have each other's keys in case of an emergency. "It's more than security—it's the voice during the day if you live alone," she said.

Another call came in. Someone needed help installing new computer software. And another, this one from a member with an old vacuum cleaner that needed a new belt.

Patrick, who had returned on his bicycle from Harris Teeter where he purchased Pauline's groceries, asked if I'd like to come with him to deliver them. Pauline, who is legally blind and lives in the basement apartment of her daughter's home, seemed happy to receive us. The aroma of the chicken filled the small kitchen.

She invited us to sit in the darkened living room for a brief chat before Patrick had to get going for his next assignment. Pauline learned about Capitol Hill Village through a friend, who saw an announcement in the *Hill Rag*, a community newspaper. "[The Village] is the best thing I've come across," she said. "What I love is when I call, I've had extended conversations with volunteers. I've had people like Patrick who are *fun*."

Pauline has difficulty getting around, but she anticipates being able to volunteer herself someday. She'd like to cofacilitate a group for other people who are visually impaired.

The list of ways Villages such as this one enrich the lives of their members or help them solve problems seems limitless. The most common request is for transportation, which Villages typically provide, often for free—to the airport, the theater, grocery shopping, or medical appointments—you name it. Home repairs are also a big need. Villages assist members by either recommending contractors whom they have vetted or by enlisting handy volunteers. At Capitol Hill, a volunteer contractor advocates for members who are negotiating home improvement contracts.

Other requests are surprising. A volunteer who enjoys sorting things might help a member who has a passion for "collecting" (i.e., hoarding) clear off the dining room table. ("We don't say 'hoarding,'" Gail explained. "Collecting is a positive word.") In all, Capitol Hill Village provided nearly three thousand services to its members in 2012, almost all by its pool of volunteers.

"You can only imagine the kinds of requests we get," said Judy Willett, executive director of Beacon Hill Village in Boston. "A member called the other day and said the vet ordered Metamucil for her cat. She didn't want to buy a whole bottle! And yes, we did have a smaller amount we could give her."

Another time, said Willett, a one-hundred-year-old member called saying she had a hankering for pizza. She couldn't possibly eat a whole one. So the staff ordered pizza the next day for lunch and took her a few slices.

Northwest Neighbors Village in Washington, DC, had an eighty-seven-year-old member whose apartment developed a terrible mold problem. The Village found her safe, temporary housing; negotiated with an elder-law attorney on her behalf; and helped her line up contractors.

While some Villages, including Beacon Hill, describe the model as a concierge service, Gail Kohn sees their role differently. She uses instead language of the heart—creating community, building relationships, staying connected, maintaining self-worth.

Sonia Crow agreed. "Part of the beauty of this is that over time, people learn to let go, to trust, to ask and not feel bad about it," she said. "I'm constantly learning things—sociologically and psychologically. There are pockets of real grace with this Village."

Grace can come when a member, living alone, has a medical problem and is soothed by hearing a friendly voice on the other end of the phone when she calls the Village. Or it can come through connections formed among people who otherwise would not meet. As part of Sonia Crow's outreach to the community, she contacted local schools to set up intergenerational relationships with members. The oldest member of Palisades Village was Miss Betty, ninety-six, who lived near a neighborhood school. The administrator thought it would be nice for the school's four-year-olds to get to know an elder in the community. Initially, the idea was for a one-time field trip to Miss Betty's home at Christmas time. She served the children cookies and milk, and together they sang holiday songs. The kids enjoyed it so much, the teachers decided to continue the relationship. Next, Miss Betty was invited to visit the children for a tea party at their school. Then came sharing green milkshakes on St. Patrick's Day, followed by an Easter egg hunt in Miss Betty's yard.

"I certainly hope that five years from now, Villages will have proliferated across the United States," said Sonia. "I've seen firsthand the place it fills in people's lives."

Whether the model succeeds in keeping people in their own homes and out of assisted living or nursing homes, as the founders hope, is too early to say. So, too, is whether it's sustainable over the long haul.

According to a 2012 survey by researchers at Rutgers University there were eighty-five Villages in the United States, with 120 more being organized. As far as socioeconomic status, nearly half of Villages were in high to middle-to-high income areas, 20 percent in middle income, and 16 percent in low to middle income areas. Some represented neighborhoods, such as Capitol Hill, while others served members in several nearby towns or in an entire town or county. Nearly 80 percent had a paid staff member. The vast majority (94 percent) of Village members nationally were white, and more than 70 percent were in the age range of sixty-five to eighty-four with nearly that many being women. Half lived alone. Fourteen percent of Village members needed assistance with personal care and nearly one-quarter with household chores.[1]

Nationally, many Villages are linked through the Village-to-Village Network, based in Boston, to share information and resources. Through webinars, the Internet, and an annual conference, they swap what they've learned about the intricacies of fundraising, establishing a nonprofit organization and board governance, budgeting, managing volunteers, and recruiting members.

Leaders of the movement are fond of saying, "If you've seen one Village, you've seen one Village." This is not a cookie cutter approach, although the early adopters have created manuals to guide emerging organizations. In my own jurisdiction, Montgomery County, Maryland, County Executive Isaiah Leggett released a blueprint for Villages in October 2010, as a way to encourage citizens to create such organizations.[2]

In an interview, Andrew Scharlach of University of California, Berkeley, a leading Village researcher, identified three primary needs the Villages fill for their members:

> The biggest advantage is that it creates a structure whereby people can access information and services in a user-friendly way. It's a single door, a single person, a single entity to call when you need help. That's number one. Number two, it provides social connection with other folks who are similarly situated. That also is an important piece. The third piece is it provides an opportunity for empowerment, an opportunity for people at

a time in life when they may be withdrawing or losing important social roles to have a meaningful role to play, to contribute to something, to create something that is theirs. A recurring mantra among Villages is they don't want to be just another social service organization, which translates as, those members don't want to be clients, they want to have some control, not only over their own well-being, but also some control over the organizations and structures that they're part of.

The Rutgers survey found a wide range of annual dues—from $25 to $948 for an individual, with discounts given for two or more members in a household. Discounts are also often given to those who can't afford the full amount. At Capitol Hill Village, 20 percent of members are low-income, although 50 percent of the larger Capitol Hill community is low-income. Some Villages find, though, that even those who are qualified for reduced dues decline to request it. "People are reluctant to ask for that," said Sonia Crow. "This is a very proud generation, extremely independent. They want to do everything themselves."

Leaders of Northwest Neighbors Village agree. According to founder and board member Frances Mahncke, her organization actually would prefer if lower-income people took the reduced dues. Many funders are only interested in supporting organizations that serve low-income people, and Villages, often located in well-to-do neighborhoods, have a hard time raising money.

Fundraising is probably the toughest obstacle to forming and maintaining a Village. While the concept sounds simple—neighbors helping neighbors—as with most alternative ways of living, a Village can be challenging to implement. What types of services can members expect? How do staff and volunteers keep from wading into problems that would be handled better by trained home health aides or social workers? How much involvement in members' lives is too much? How do you prevent volunteer burnout? Who will coordinate the community? How will decisions be made? How much will membership cost? Should there be a sliding scale—and if so, is it based on the honor system? Will all ages be welcome to join, or will it be age-restricted? How do you set up a tax-exempt nonprofit? And so on. Villages typically take two years or more to establish, once there is a core of committed founders.

Other than office space, the biggest line item is salary for a director; most Villages find it too difficult to function solely with volunteers. Northwest Neighbors began by passing a Blackberry between volunteer coordinators each day—an unworkable plan. They have since hired a director who works out of a small office donated to the organization by a nonprofit assisted living center.

Villages pay their operating expenses through a mix of dues, grants, and fundraising events or appeals. "So far, the model is viable but not sustainable," said Gail Kohn. Her goal is for Capitol Hill Village to be self-sufficient, but in 2012, less than half of its $327,000 in annual revenue came from member dues, with the balance coming from contributions, grants, and special events.

At least one Village in the Washington, DC, area has taken a different approach. Bannockburn Neighbors Assisting Neighbors (NAN) is an all-volunteer, intergenerational organization formed officially in 2009 as a simple and low-key way to support each other. "Our board has a strong preference for focusing on services and activities rather than administration or bookkeeping," explained NAN president Miriam Kelty. "If you have a paid person, you have to pay worker's comp, and you need to generate a substantial amount of money and that would change the nature of our organization."

Bannockburn is an older neighborhood in Bethesda, Maryland, made up of 450 households knitted together by a strong sense of community. The neighborhood was built on a bankrupt golf course and the original clubhouse remains a central gathering place where NAN members can meet.

Early on they created a survey to find out both what people's needs were and whether they'd like to volunteer. The survey was distributed by block coordinators, who were assisted with follow-up by neighborhood teens. The survey asked if respondents either needed help or were willing to help with errands, transportation, basic computer assistance, equipment loans (from wheelchairs to infant car seats), household chores, friendly visits, and yard help. As with most Villages, far more people are willing to help others than to request help for themselves.

To try to make sure no one falls through the cracks, each block coordinator is assigned fifteen or so households to stay in touch with, making sure that anyone who would like help receives it.

NAN also organizes events in the community, drawing on their neighbors' expertise to offer programs such as a container gardening workshop led by a master gardener or a talk on aging and memory led by a speech therapist. To foster intergenerational friendship NAN initiated a Wise Elder project, which pairs elders with high school students to build a mentor relationship and produce an oral history. The final presentations are given to the community in the clubhouse. The teens have produced photo albums, PowerPoint presentations, genealogical investigations, and other creative projects together with their "Wise Elder." "It's worked out very nicely," said Miriam. "The school system shows up, the kids bring their families, the older people bring theirs."

Most Villages, though, are not all-volunteer, and Scharlach agrees that long-term sustainability is a big question. "There are a couple [of Villages] that already have closed their doors or decided not to open their doors because the energy dissipated," he said. One challenge is financial, when projected numbers of members do not pan out or members who do join do not renew. "My sense is that members join either because there is something immediate they get out of it, or because of the future promise that there will be services there when they need them. One challenge for Villages is to have programs and ways of involving members that are meaningful in the now, not just in the future. Some Villages have done a better job than others."

At the same time, he said, "You're creating a nonprofit organization, a business entity, and like any new business, a bunch will fail even if you've got a great idea, either because of marketing, or your business plan is not as solid as you'd hoped, or you don't have the technical know-how to make it all work. These are not experts who are coming together to do this; they are well-meaning, committed, caring, excited, local residents. Having the economic and technical resources to make it work takes a bunch of energy. It takes sustaining that energy over the long term."

Charismatic leadership is key, he said, both in terms of a director and a board or active committee members willing to share the load. Such leaders don't necessarily come from the neighborhood. I was surprised to learn that Gail Kohn does not live in the Capitol Hill neighborhood, for example. She sees being an outsider as an advantage. She does not know the local history or stories, rather, she is on the receiving end, learning from the Village members, which is where she wants to be.

She and her husband live in my hometown of Takoma Park, Maryland, which straddles Washington. They moved into a remodeled basement apartment in their son and daughter-in-law's house—another way to choose to age. Gail invited me over one day to continue our discussion of Villages. A wide staircase led up from the apartment to the rest of the house, an open invitation for her grandchildren to come down and hang out. Downsizing from a big house to this apartment was both challenging and liberating, she said.

In theory (and according to her paycheck), Gail worked thirty-two hours a week for Capitol Hill Village. But even when she's home, she's on call. She answers her work cell phone twenty-four hours a day, seven days a week, in order to meet any emergencies that arise with members. Gail proactively takes steps to support members whose physical or cognitive needs make aging in place a challenge, if not impossible. The Village has helped arrange personal care for forty members, allowing them to remain in their homes. Capitol Hill also partners with a medical house-call program, where a doctor or nurse practitioner comes to a member's house. Medicare and other insurance programs cover the cost, she added.

Capitol Hill Village also developed a medical advocate program, where trained volunteers accompany members to doctor's appointments. "The advocates do three things," Gail explained. "Work with the member on their expectations for the appointment and help them hone questions for the doctor, go with them to the appointment and take notes, and review the upshot with the doctor." Advocates are encouraged not to directly ask questions during the appointment unless the member has forgotten what to ask.

Despite the group's best efforts, she said, "We've lost a number of members who need, for safety reasons, to move to assisted living or a nursing home. They're leaving because they are cognitively impaired, or some have physical disabilities and are sick of dealing with the kitchen on one floor and the bathroom on another."

Always one to push the envelope, Gail now is working on a new vision to meet the needs of such members. She'd like an intergenerational day care center for both children and elders who need assistance. She'd like to build a small home in the neighborhood (see Chapter 16), where people who need nursing home-level care could move and still be part of their long-time community. She envisions a mix of housing and services and income levels, all strands woven together to keep their community tightly knit and intact.

☙❧

It was five fifteen in the morning and I was sitting on my porch with a thermos of coffee in mild September darkness. I was waiting for Gail to pick me up so that I could tag along as she took a member to a medical appointment. From my porch, I saw an SUV stop down the street. I strolled down the block and saw Gail fiddling with her cell phone. She laughed when I pointed out that she was at the wrong house. "It's my cataracts," she said, explaining that she'd misread the house number.

Gail is a tough, good-natured woman. Tough in the way of being determined to get back to sculling every morning on the Potomac River despite painful osteoarthritis of the knees. Tough in the way of driving in the dark to unfamiliar neighborhoods in service to a worthy cause. She's in her sixties and realizes she might want to plan for her own retirement before too many years go by. She's spent a lifetime working in eldercare, including being the administrator of a large nonprofit continuing care retirement community in Maryland.

"I'm overqualified for this," she said of her job as director of Capitol Hill Village. "But I love it. It's fun."

We wound our way through our town and crossed over into Washington, heading south on North Capitol Street. The sight of the Capitol dome glowing against the deep blue of the pre-dawn sky still gives me a thrill, even though I've lived here most of my life.

Gail turned in front of the grand edifice of Union Station and slowly made her way to our destination. Luckily there was little traffic as we stopped frequently to peer at street signs.

We were taking a member, Elizabeth, up to Baltimore for an MRI at Johns Hopkins University Hospital. I learned that she'd had undiagnosed fiery pain in her head. Elizabeth emerged from her townhouse along with her sister, Joan, who had come down from Philadelphia to offer moral support. At first I thought it was Joan whom we'd come to help. It was she who used a cane and walked painfully down the steps. She climbed into the SUV with obvious difficulty. Elizabeth seemed healthier. Both women were short and heavy-set with dark hair. Joan was a cancer survivor and a PhD clinical social worker whose specialty is children. She sat in back with me.

Once settled in the front seat next to Gail, Elizabeth seemed morose and worried. She had spent six hours in the emergency room at Georgetown University Medical Center the day before and left without feeling any relief. Gail asked her what happened in the ER.

"This is making me anxious to think about," Elizabeth said. We steered the conversation elsewhere.

As we headed up the Baltimore-Washington Parkway, the sky faded to morning. Gail wended her way through downtown Baltimore. She let us off in front of the massive Johns Hopkins complex, where I retrieved a wheelchair for Joan. Elizabeth was impressed with how friendly hospital employees were—the guard, the receptionist. The walk to the MRI center in the basement was a long one. Despite the hospital's stellar reputation, the basement seemed dingy and unappealing.

The woman behind the big desk in the MRI office was friendly and professional. She gave Elizabeth the usual forms to complete. Elizabeth looked at us and wondered aloud if she should take the Ativan she'd brought along to reduce her anxiety. Neither Joan nor I responded.

Before long, Elizabeth's name was called, and she disappeared down a long hall with a young woman dressed in scrubs. Joan called to her sister to come get her, whenever she was needed. Gail arrived, having parked the car, and immediately began wrapping her arthritic knees in ice bags she'd lugged along. She joked and didn't complain, but obviously she was hurting.

Elizabeth emerged within minutes looking despondent. "They won't do it," she said. It turned out she has implanted in her ears some small tubes that could cause the magnetic apparatus in the MRI to go haywire. Having an

MRI, she was told, was potentially dangerous. Elizabeth was upset that the doctor had told her to come, even though he was aware of the implants.

We gathered our belongings—apples, knitting, notebook, Gail's ice pack, coffee thermoses—and trudged back through the dingy halls far sooner than we had imagined. Elizabeth was upset. As we walked, she used her cell phone to call the doctor and miraculously reached him. He was apologetic. He thought the MRI people were mistaken, but it was too late to make the test happen that day.

Back in the car we climbed. On the return trip, Elizabeth visibly brightened, despite her disappointment. Her mood had shifted from morose and anxious to loquacious, from tentative and insecure to resolute as she expounded about politics (our favorite local sport).

I asked her about the Village. "I heard about it for years, but didn't think I needed it," she said. "Then I realized it's not about need, but support. The vision is to fulfill the interests of any member who wants to stay in their house. You can see how it saved my life here."

Elizabeth has lived on Capitol Hill for forty years. "It's always been a community-oriented neighborhood," she said. "We used to have a babysitting co-op. Now traffic is horrendous, and a lot of the young people don't give a hoot about the community."

Gail gently interjected that many of their volunteers are younger. "One brings her one-year-old along and that's fun for people," she said. In fact, one-third of the Village's 180 volunteers are thirty years old or younger, many of them tech-savvy. "Although our best tech person is seventy," she added.

After we said our good-byes to Elizabeth and Joan, Gail smiled. "We did good work," she said. I realized she was right. Success, by Gail's lights, didn't mean completing the task of Elizabeth getting an MRI. It's not something you can check off a to-do list. Success instead meant being in companionship with someone who was hurting and helping shoulder a burden that clearly felt too heavy to bear. I was just an observer in this drama, but I got it. And if even for just a few hours, I felt privileged to be along for the ride.

CHAPTER 4

Cohousing

Creating Community
from the Ground Up

Imagine living in a community where you know all your neighbors. The houses are designed and sited in a way that encourages friendly encounters while at the same time maintaining personal privacy. Friends in this close-knit neighborhood frequently dine together in the common house, an area with a commercial kitchen and a large dining area, big enough to hold all who wish to come. Some folks organize spontaneous get-togethers in the large den to watch sports or have cocktails. People share lawnmowers, tools, even washers and dryers if they wish, because they decided everyone does not need to own every item a household uses from time to time.

This may sound utopian, but it's everyday life for people who have chosen cohousing.

Perhaps more than those of any other living arrangement, proponents of cohousing consider themselves part of a movement, one that aims to create intentional communities and liberate people from isolation and loneliness. "I can't imagine not living in cohousing," said Ann Zabaldo, in her early sixties, who lives in Takoma Village in Washington, DC. (To be clear, Takoma Village is a cohousing community, not a Village as described in the previous chapter.) "What would that be like? It would be akin to living on a desert island. It's like the old saying—the worst day in cohousing beats the best day at the beach."

Oz Ragland, fifty-four, like Ann, is a national leader in the cohousing movement. He recently shifted his focus to shared housing. He and his wife and a few others now live next door to the Songaia Cohousing Community they helped to found north of Seattle. Oz said the appeal of living in community goes far beyond saving money on housing costs. "Shared housing and cohousing have created wonderful social environments for older folk and younger folk," he said. "You're no longer sitting there alone, eating alone, [spending] most of your time alone."

Cohousing was the brainchild of Danish architect Jan Gudmand-Hoyer, who came up with the idea of a more supportive living environment in 1964.

It took more than a decade for the first cohousing community to be built in Denmark, where the model is now an accepted part of the housing mix. Cohousing was brought to the United States by architect and spousal team Charles Durrett and Kathryn McCamant in the mid-1980s. As Durrett wrote, "The Danes, like Americans, value the ideals of individualism and self-sufficiency . . . [cohousing] residents aren't so much living in a mutually dependent relationship as they are engaged in a mutually beneficial partnership."[1]

As of April 2013 there were over one hundred completed communities and a roughly equal number in various stages of formation in thirty-seven states and Washington, DC, according to the directory of the Cohousing Association of the United States. Four were listed as disbanded or dormant.

Unlike a commune, where members jointly own property, cohousing communities are generally set up as condominiums as far as legal ownership and structure. "Some [communes] are in much more utopian communities that are living some kind of political agenda—income sharing or following some kind of vision," explained Oz. "Communes have income sharing by definition." Cohousing's only agenda, he said, is to nurture a strong sense of community.

Each person or family purchases (or in some cases rents) their own unit, which has everything a normal household would have—a full kitchen, living room, bedrooms. These units are linked to large common spaces, designed to suit the community.

Durrett identifies six characteristics that distinguish cohousing from other living arrangements:

- Participatory process. Residents are involved in the planning and design of the community.
- Deliberate neighborhood design. The design encourages community; think front porches not rear decks.
- Extensive common facilities. Unlike a condominium party room, cohousing's common spaces are meant for everyday use by the whole community.
- Complete resident management. Residents make decisions together, typically in a consensus style.
- Non-hierarchical structure. There are no formal leadership roles.
- Separate income sources. Residents do not earn their income from the community.[2]

Cohousing may be found in urban, rural, or small town areas, and the individual units can be market-rate or affordable, or both within one community. They may be built from the ground up or in renovated space, such as Swan's Market in Oakland, California, which was built in an abandoned city market. In Denver, a block of 1940s townhouses is being retrofitted to make a cohousing community. Turtle Farm Cohousing Community in Granger, Iowa, aims to sustain an organic farm on its property. Columbia Ecovillage, with thirty-seven condominium units, is one of six urban cohousing communities in Portland, Oregon.

Each cohousing community is unique, reflecting its founding group. "We shouldn't get too bogged down in the physical and design aspects of cohousing," was a comment on a cohousing listserv. "Building coho trailer parks, slowly converting apartment buildings, organically changing neighborhoods—these should all be part of the mix."[3]

Most cohousing is not age-restricted, and many residents prefer the blend of young and old living in community together. Grace Kim, a Seattle architect, is a strong believer in multigenerational cohousing. "For me, the interest and attraction in cohousing is the intergenerationality of it," she said. "Part of it is a cultural thing—we're losing respect for elders. From that standpoint, cohousing allows there to be a better understanding and relationship. It allows old people to mentor or provide guidance and assistance if society doesn't give value to the things they have to contribute in later years. I feel cohousing is very aware of that and embraces that."

Others are ready for the quiet and calm that comes with living with their peers as they age. A few senior cohousing communities have been developed, and more are on the drawing board.

Many cohousing units are sold at market rate and can be pricey. The units at Takoma Village reflect the housing costs of Washington, DC, one of the highest real estate markets in the nation. An 820-square foot, two-bedroom apartment, for example, sells for more than $300,000.

But some cohousing communities seek to maintain at least some affordable units. Boulder Creek, one of the oldest cohousing communities, was organized in 1987 and is committed to affordability, including an option to have reduced monthly fees in exchange for more community participation, such as cooking a group meal. It also offers prospective community members the option of renting first, to test the waters, and then buying if it's a good fit. Svaboda Court in Portland, Oregon, is a cohousing community made up entirely of affordable units, available to people who earn in the $25,000 to $45,000 range. In New Mexico, Sand River Cohousing (originally called ElderGrace) was developed by the Santa Fe Community Housing Trust. Units for those who meet income guidelines are as low as $80,000. Jim Hannan, who helped design and develop Sand River, worries that over time, those affordable units will be sold at market rate once the original owners are gone. The city of Santa Fe partially owns the below-market units, and Hannan wonders if they are committed to affordability.

On the other hand, he said, "The thing about cohousing, these are committed people, a cut above your average homeowners association. They are politically active, usually environmentalists, so they are the kind of person who knows how the system works. If they decided it was an important value to keep some units affordable, my sense is they could mobilize a little bit and go before city council and come up with a memorandum to make it happen."

As Hannan suggests, a strong environmental ethic is another hallmark of many cohousing communities. For example, the first senior cohousing community to share a site with multigenerational cohousing was initiated by a group of environmentalists in Denmark in 1995. "The goal was to make the houses as ecologically sustainable as possible without sacrificing basic comfort," wrote Durrett.[4]

Cohousing communities generally use less than half the amount of land of a typical subdivision for a comparable number of households, and residences are significantly smaller. The average size of new homes in the United States is more than 2,300 square feet; cohousing units average roughly half that amount.[5]

Community members tend to be comfortable with smaller households in exchange for the large common spaces. "Most people who move to cohousing are downsizing," said Ann Zabaldo. "They want less responsibility as far as physical upkeep."

Cohousing communities often place a high value on energy-efficiency and environmentally-friendly construction. Members use 25 percent as much energy as the average American household, and they drive cars 25 percent less. Takoma Village has a geothermal heating and cooling system, for example, and a two-bedroom unit has an average monthly utility bill of $75. Eastern Village nearby has won awards for its "green" building and includes a rooftop garden. Liberty Village in Frederick County, Maryland, has roomy duplexes sited on land that includes fifteen acres of meadow, woods, and wetlands. The entire community received training for "Bay-Wise Certification" from a master gardener, meaning their practices promote restoration of the Chesapeake Bay. Rain gardens and wetlands control runoff, helping keep pollutants from reaching the Bay.

Although I found no one who thought cohousing was the domain of people with a liberal political persuasion, the cohousing residents I interviewed fit that description. "Certainly there are religious groups who decide to live communally that can be very conservative in terms of 'family values,'" said Marty of Sand River. "Cohousing I think would work whatever your political point of view. However when you think about the commune movement in the 1960s it was full of flaming liberals. There's a history of cooperation and communal living in the liberal wing of the country that is not so present in the conservative side of things. When I think of political conservatives I think of people who believe in rugged independence, and 'I'm the captain of my fate,' whereas we're a little less like that."

Marty was drawn to cohousing out of a desire to have community and to live in an affordable, energy-efficient home, all of which she found at Sand River. Earlier in her life, as a school teacher and single mom with an adopted daughter from Central America, she experienced the loneliness of suburban life. Although she was glad to have the summers off to be with her daughter, she said, "It was so lonely. There I was on this street, sort of a bedroom community, and everybody else was at work, and I was home alone with this little person, going crazy. I just remember how that was—that's not how I want to spend my retirement, just cooped up in a house and there's no one to do anything with. And knowing I'd have to get in a car and drive to an organized event. [Here], if I'm feeling under the weather or upset about something, I can walk out my door."

Jim Hannan said cohousing is ideal for single people like Marty or those who are introverts. "Depending on your personality and how your life looks, it might be a much better way to live," he said. "If you're introverted and shy, and your best friend moved to Phoenix, well, now you're living with twenty-seven potential friends at [Sand River] who are easily accessible. You're twenty feet from neighbors across the way. If you go to the common house once or twice during the day, the mailbox is there, or you go in and make coffee or watch a movie. I think life is about probability—the key to successful social life is to maximize positive human connections." Extroverts, he said, might be able to create those connections on their own; introverts may need more help.

♾

Takoma Village, near my home, is a large U-shaped development in a neighborhood that straddles DC and Maryland.

The wider community has a diverse mix of incomes and races and is a short walk to the subway, restaurants, farmers' market, and shops. Takoma Village describes itself as "an eclectic community of 68 adults from several cultural backgrounds and many fields of interest, and 21 children, aged 3 months to 90 years," as well as four dogs and many cats.[6]

As with all cohousing, the common spaces are designed to suit the community. At the bottom of the U, there is a large kitchen and dining area, a living room with a fireplace where a dozen or more people can watch the Olympics, election returns, or movies; a large toddler playroom filled with an inviting array of toys that opens to an outdoor playground; a "Take It or Leave It" corner where people swap belongings; a fitness room; workshop; an office with computer and fax machine; and a small room where teens can play Wii and other games.

Peter and Sharyn, who are now in their sixties, moved to Takoma Village in 2000. They had been living in a single-family house a few miles away in Silver Spring and had both been interested for many years in some form of cooperative living. Sharyn had once envisioned buying a house or apartment building with friends, where they would live together and run an on-site tutoring program. Peter was drawn to cohousing back in the 1980s. Eventually, they discovered the group organizing Takoma Village and decided this was the community they'd been looking for. They bought a two-bedroom townhouse; options range from one-bedroom apartments to four-bedroom townhouses, all facing a common grassy area with room for garden plots.

Thirteen years later, they're glad they put down roots. "I foresee us staying here until some life change happens," said Peter. They each have found their niche in the community. Sharyn has helped with managing the guest quarters and with community celebrations, while Peter, the more gregarious, is active on many committees and has held leadership positions.

"I like that people are supporting each other and reach out to each other," said Sharyn. "I love the fact that we celebrate holidays together and have respect for each other's traditions. I like that there's a sense of community around the children."

Near Seattle Oz Ragland contrasts his own childhood, living in a nuclear family with a mother who had mental health issues, with that of his own son who grew up at Songaia Cohousing. "Here in my community, my son was a single child but lived with twelve other kids and twenty other adults," said Oz. "He got to see these models of different ways of being."

The design and intentionality of cohousing encourages friendship across generations. "It is a place where you can be a grandparent to kids who aren't yours, or an uncle or aunt," said Oz. "I see that in our community. We have some elderly folks who have certain kids who visit with them all the time."

He gives the example of Amelia, who as a little girl always came and had breakfast with Nancy, an older woman with whom she could hang out before school since her parents had to go to work early. "Giving older people a purpose for being and a way to give and to contribute is so important," he said. "The most active contributors in our community have been the seniors."

At Eastern Village, the older members have formed an ad hoc group called the Sages, who get together to discuss topics of interest and to socialize.

Governing by Consensus

While cohousing communities pride themselves in having strong neighborly bonds, that doesn't mean they are easy to organize or to govern. They generally require a substantial capital investment either for new construction or major renovation. That money usually comes from a pool of founding members who pre-purchase their units. "One of the problems about cohousing is that it's so difficult to create one and they're so expensive that they fail to get done," said Oz. After an initial burst of enthusiasm, the complexities of design and construction and the inevitable compromises that must be made due to cost constraints can dampen commitment.

While some might embrace this lifestyle, it runs counter to what many consider a distinct part of American culture: cohousing requires forsaking some autonomy for strong community. As Silvine Farnell, a member of the group that founded Silver Sage senior cohousing in Boulder, Colorado, put it, "To live in cohousing you have to let go of a lot of control, there's a surrendering. I'm drawn to the growth that comes out of this surrender, and still, sometimes I ask myself, 'What am I getting into?'"[7]

That surrender is embodied in a consensus style of governing. Consensus, for the uninitiated, is a method to reach agreement, especially on important decisions. It allows for everyone's voice to be heard and considered and for disagreements to be hashed out until everyone can at least live with the result, even if they're not thrilled with it.

The problem with consensus, said Peter of Takoma Village, is that "it's too easy for one person to drag things out." As a result, some members feel "it's easier not to get involved." Common areas of disagreement in cohousing communities include equitable sharing of work around the place, whether or not to charge for the guestroom, whether cooking common meals should be required or voluntary, and so on. Some cohousing communities solve the work-sharing by hiring outsiders to take care of landscaping or cleaning common spaces. At Takoma Village, residents share many of the chores, "but the work is not evenly divided," said Peter. "Some people, it rubs them horrendously that some do almost nothing." The bylaws of Takoma Village state that you are expected to spend some time serving the community and if you don't, you must pay extra, but this policy is not enforced, he said.

Sharyn added that the decision-making process is a real problem as far as she is concerned. "It's taken a year to consense on an area rug for the common house," she said.

David Wann wrote in his book *Reinventing Community* about what many would see as this downside of cohousing. He described a beautiful fall day in Colorado with a hot game of football—Broncos versus the Raiders—on the tube. But it's the day for a community meeting to discuss a contentious issue on how tasks get done and what is considered essential versus nonessential work. "Fasten your seat belts, ladies and gentlemen, this could be a turbulent ride," he wrote. "By comparison it might be less stressful to spend the afternoon balancing the checkbook, carrying heavy boxes, or having a root canal.

"Why do we do it? Why do we swim upstream like 10,000 salmon when hitching a ride down the mainstream currents of suburban or apartment life might require so much less exertion? Why are we working so hard to invent a new, improved American Dream?"[8]

Others answer this question by saying that consensus is a valuable way to strengthen the community. "There are a couple of values that cohousing represents that are important," said Ed, who lives with his wife Joan at Eastern Village, a cohousing community not far from Takoma Village. Noting that he had been a professional mediator, Ed appreciates consensus. "Consensus decision making really is a form of mediation," he said. "It's an important experiment for America in how to make decisions and it's an opportunity to sharpen skills.

"A lot of people feel alienated in life. It's useful to find ways for people to live in community. The relationships you develop are nice. We have a genuinely fond feeling toward the people here."

Catherine of ElderSpirit in Abingdon, Virginia, also appreciates the consensus method and feels it can lead to better decisions—a case of the whole being wiser than the sum of its parts. "Everybody's opinion is considered important, and everybody needs to be heard," she said. "The decisions lead to some compromises that are often better than the one put forward that would have been approved by the majority."

For example, the original architectural design for ElderSpirit had the Spirit Center, which serves as a chapel and meditation room, near the Common House. But they did not have enough money to build it during the first phase of construction.

Once people had moved in, many did not like the planned location. Some realized they'd be looking out on a building rather than at their neighbors. They convinced the others to build the Spirit Center at the end of the property. "I was among those who wanted the original architectural plan," said

Catherine. "We ended up changing the plan, and I think everybody is happy with it now."

According to the Cohousing Association website, the key is to use consensus sparingly, for big decisions that are meant to last. "For a group deciding its mission, values, or high-level policies—all intended to endure for future generations—taking the time to develop consensus among all members is worth the effort. Deciding what to have for lunch—a decision that lasts only through dessert—is not worth the effort to achieve consensus."[9]

All that said, there is no law that a cohousing community must use consensus. Ann Zabaldo notes that consensus was never part of cohousing in Denmark, the birthplace of the model. "I'm encouraging other forms of governance," she said. "We've used [consensus] here but it's a lot of work. I don't think it has to be like that."

Senior Cohousing

In the remote southwestern tip of Virginia, Dene Peterson, a former Sister of Loretto, a progressive community of Catholic nuns, organized ElderSpirit, one of the first senior cohousing communities in the nation. "My family thought I was off my gourd for doing this," she said.

But Dene had a clear mission. "I wanted to show that different things can be done," she said. "With the baby boomers, aging will take its proper place."

The community is guided by a vision of living simply and sustainably, recognizing the role of spirituality and supporting each other through the end of life. It welcomes people fifty-five and older of all faiths and income levels, with sixteen units dedicated as affordable rental housing, and thirteen for purchase at market rate. That commitment to include low-income people presents ongoing challenges for ElderSpirit, but Dene and other founding members don't waver.

"The income mix is really important," said Catherine, eighty-three, also a former Sister. "People who have enough money have many choices of how to live. People without money don't have many choices. . . . In neighborhoods where everyone is low income they don't have influence over what happens in those areas. That's an awful way to live. Here, they feel safe, they trust their neighbors, they don't lock their door. Knowing and trusting our neighbors makes life a whole lot easier."

Dene's unit is 760 square feet, with high ceilings and plenty of sunlight. Each unit has a front porch and a window over the kitchen sink, looking out over the common grounds. Many people have gardens, and each household does its own landscaping.

Once a week, people gather in the Common House to share a meal. In addition to a commercial kitchen and large dining room, the Common House has two guest bedrooms; a laundry; a library; a game room; a large, well-lit art studio; and meeting space. People square dance, discuss community chores, and hold forums on such topics as "How do you feel about asking for help?" There's exercise equipment and an outdoor grill.

On the other end of the property is the octagonal Spirit House, where residents hold vespers, Sunday services, meditation, and yoga practice. People are encouraged to connect with the wider community and to volunteer in the town of Abingdon, including at a Head Start center nearby.

Dene, who said she is "opposed to nursing homes," is convinced that with home health care and housekeeping services, most members of their community will never have to move. "I did this because I didn't want to die alone," she said. If someone does have to go to a nursing home, ElderSpirit members are committed to visiting them regularly and keeping them as part of the community as best they can.

As one founding resident, Monica, reflected, on why she appreciates senior cohousing, "You have neighbors wanting to live in an intentional community, who want to participate in common meals, who have concern for the environment, and who have an interest in late-life spirituality—who, if you're ill, will help with meals and transportation. You can usually find someone to visit with. It's a proactive way to plan for older, more frail, years so that a community of friendship can be built for as long as possible."

Senior cohousing offers residents key features of healthy aging: a strong social network and a great deal of purpose through opportunities to serve the community—what Charles Durrett describes as "an exit strategy where they plan for and get the most out of their last 20 years—without being a burden to their children, without having to completely rely on the government, without compromising their own potential for happiness."[10] Unlike intergenerational cohousing where much of the attention is focused on the children and common meals can be boisterous affairs, choosing to live among peers gives older people more peace and a chance to reflect on the spiritual challenges of growing frailer and facing the end of life.

ElderSpirit has an intentionality about aging that is refreshing. The community holds a monthly meeting to discuss issues such as respect for aging, American culture's "adoration of youth," and aging as a life stage that is respectable and enjoyable, a time to be appreciated and to make a contribution to the world. Catherine calls this a time of "conscious aging." Unafraid to talk about the inevitability of dying, she reflected, "One might have more time for prayer, reading, and meditation, and it's good to have that time preparing to meet God."

When you turn eighty, said Carol, another ElderSpirit resident, something shifts inside. "You're looking closer to death and to having some comfort. That subject is very important. You're winnowing down ambition, which is simpler and leaves you more content.

"The gain? You slow down and smell the daisies. There's time to do things and have more appreciation of the natural world and people. It's hard to let yourself slow down. It's kind of a spiritual challenge to allow yourself to slow down and to use more wisdom and less strength."

ElderSpirit's spiritual component is stronger than most cohousing communities. Although founded by Catholic nuns, people of many faiths live there, including Protestants, Quakers, and Buddhists. Those who wish to can take turns leading weekly prayer service. "The summer solstice celebration was well-attended," said Dene. "People respect each other's spiritual practices and beliefs."

The biggest challenges are less spiritual than practical, and some question whether the commitment to provide affordable rentals is worth it.

Dene developed the business plan for the community. Her previous work had been as parish administrator of the Newman Center at University of Michigan, where she led a large capital campaign. "I learned how to raise money and to sell people on ideas and to take risks," she said. "I learned what a million was. And what construction and development was. I'm entrepreneurial—but only when it's a nonprofit. Service is the bottom line."

Dene and a group of friends formed the nonprofit Trailview Development Company and put together what eventually grew to a $3.6 million package of loans and grants. They purchased 3.7 acres for the twenty-nine homes and common property. Part of their financing came in the form of government loans for construction of affordable housing, which came with considerable strings attached.

Both renters and homeowners whom I interviewed say they don't feel a dichotomy or social division between the two groups, a process Dene nudged along by making sure renters held leadership roles from the beginning. "I'm very aware of prejudice against poor people," she said, and she's worked to guard against it at ElderSpirit.

Still, the process of preserving affordable rental units is fraught. "Affordable housing, because of the loan documents, is a challenge to community building," said Carol. "We didn't come here to fuss about finances. We came to build a community. In spite of that, I feel it will work. But I doubt it will be replicated."

During my visit, the community was in turmoil over a woman who had rented there for three years. A government auditor noticed that the woman now made 50.45 percent of the median income, just a smidgeon (less than $100 annually) above the 50 percent cutoff. ElderSpirit was told they had to remedy the situation—meaning the woman had to move out—or pay back the $178,000 Federal Home Loan grant they'd received for construction. The dilemma divided the community.

Even as they dealt with this difficult situation, residents spoke warmly of their lives there. Carolyn, sixty-seven, a local woman, is a self-described black sheep of her family. Her daughter discovered ElderSpirit on the Internet and encouraged Carolyn to move there. "I know everybody in the county anyway, and I know everybody here," she said. "Every member of my family thinks it's the greatest thing. They're glad I've settled here. I like helping other people. I love cooking someone a meal or sitting with them or doing some laundry. Everyone here is appreciative and no one takes advantage." Even as a younger member of the community, Carolyn, who had dealt with major medical issues, said she appreciates that people are not afraid to talk about death.

One of ElderSpirit's signature programs is informal care coordination. Each resident has a care coordinator, either a spouse or another member of ElderSpirit, who acts as an advocate should you have medical problems. Care coordinators find out what you need or want—help with meals at your home, invitations to dinner, transportation, dog walking—and reach out to let others know how they can help.

ElderSpirit residents also pitch in by volunteering with the Hospitality Committee, the Membership Committee, the Spirituality Committee, and so on. "It's complicated but it works very well," said Catherine. "It's not like in a [Catholic] religious community, where a Superior is in charge. That's fine, but it's hierarchical. I think it's better this way."

At the same time, it's challenging, to take the time and effort to consult with the community, rather than making decisions yourself. This is clearly not a lifestyle that would appeal to everyone. But the trade-off in having a close supportive network of people around you is worth it, say those who have chosen to live in an intentional community like ElderSpirit.

Linda and Roger, sixty-four and seventy-one respectively, had a tough decision as far as moving there. They were both involved in community and church (she's Lutheran, he's Catholic) in Illinois, when they read a news story about ElderSpirit. Their son lives not far away in Knoxville, Tennessee, so they decided to come to the region and check it out. ElderSpirit was then a sea of slabs, mud, and wood. "I remember walking through mud—not the most encouraging first glimpse," said Roger. "When we met Catherine and Dene, that convinced me."

As a former priest, he had lived in community before. He is now an active member of the men's group, which has breakfast together every Friday, as well as a men's prayer group. He also developed a spiritual quest for residents, taking advantage of the Creeper Trail that runs for miles behind the property.

Linda said the committee work can be time-consuming and even get in the way of other things that are important to her—hobbies, church activities, even forming friendships. She appreciates that the community also has a lot of fun together—movies, talent nights, joke nights, exercise, common meals, as well as spontaneous outings, to a winery or sculpture garden.

I asked Catherine what qualities are important for someone to fit in well at ElderSpirit. "The desire to cooperate with other people," she said. "The desire to be helpful and to receive help, to have an interest in spiritual things, to be willing to do work in the community.

"So many people are left alone in their older years. We need to try to do better. My family still has extended family helping older people. But a lot of people don't have that. I think [cohousing] is one good solution. So far it works. If we have a lot of old, sick people we'll have to see."

☙❧

At the other end of the senior cohousing spectrum is Glacier Circle in Davis, a prosperous town in northern California. Ellen Coppock organized the community in 2002, and construction was completed in 2006. Unlike ElderSpirit, which sought a mixed income group of many faiths, Ellen and her husband reached out to their own church network to share the last chapter together. "We took the Unitarian address book and sent out about thirty or forty invitations to people we thought might be interested and would fit in," she said. "We have all gotten along very well—we're all quite liberal politically, and we have shared values."

The key, she said, is shared values, no matter what they are. "If we had a fundamentalist Christian in our group that wouldn't be good, because our values are tremendously different," she said. "However, there are other people that we would welcome for sure. We have Jewish neighbors that we asked, and they considered it. They didn't because of their dietary reasons, and that would have been a problem, but otherwise they would have fit."

Glacier Circle is tiny—just eight units—because the only piece of land they could find in Davis was less than one acre. All but one homeowner was able to purchase their house outright, from the sale of their former home; the one person who is an exception has a mortgage. All members continue to attend the Unitarian church where they met. Glacier Circle has a waiting list, and Ellen is optimistic they will stay full.

Their challenge, though, is the same as many age-restricted communities—attracting people young enough to help out the others. Ellen ticks off the ages of Glacier Circle members: "Four of us are eighty-six and there are three ninety-year-olds. Pretty quick, we're all going to start dying off. Nobody talks about it, but we all have it in the back of our mind."

For now, enough continue to drive to help transport the others. Unlike most cohousing, they hire a chef to come prepare the common meal three times a week and also hire someone to help clean the common areas. They're considering hiring a shared chauffeur, as time goes on. In the meantime, Davis has an excellent bus system.

Ellen believes cohousing helps people stay independent longer than they otherwise would. She points to one of their members who has mobility problems. People help push her wheelchair or provide transportation. "She is far better off than in an assisted living place at the moment and much happier," she said. "She knows all of us and we all love her."

As for intergenerational cohousing, the concept holds no appeal for Ellen. "Soon after we moved in we were invited to [another cohousing community] and they have a lot of children," she said. "Nobody sat with us, everybody had their own family to take care of, and afterwards, the program was to sit and watch the kids play. That was fine for one evening, but it wasn't fine for all the time. But they're all very nice."

On an electronic listserv for cohousing communities around the nation, there have been lively discussions about the pros and cons of multigenerational versus senior cohousing. The answer seems clear: both choices have value and appeal to different people. Two cohousing communities in Boulder, Colorado, may have hit on the ideal solution: Silver Sage Village, a senior cohousing community, was built within walking distance of Wild Sage for people of all ages.

At Silver Sage, said Margaret, who lives there with her husband, the agreement is that each person is expected to be independent, health-wise. "We are each expected to provide for our own needs," she said. "We do take each other to doctor's appointments. We keep watch if someone has an acute health care crisis." When a member of the community became gravely ill, he had live-in help, went on hospice, and died at home, as he wished.

Ann Zabaldo, sixty-one, is committed to living at the multigenerational Takoma Village. But if she were to leave, she would seek out a senior cohousing community. "I'm ready to move on to whatever this stage is about," she said, "and a community better off financially as opposed to when you're raising kids. I'd like to be able to travel together. Here, there's not a big budget for social activities.

"As people get older, it gets harder to hear," she continued. "I'm getting ready for peace and quiet—which can be hard at dinnertime [because of the children]. My attention is turning to the next stage of life. Since seniors do so much work around here, I wonder if we're obfuscating the time for conversation. How do you want your death to go? It's hardly ever a topic of conversation."

Whether a cohousing community is multigenerational or senior, its willingness to assist members if they grow vulnerable and frail depends somewhat on the agreements made early on, but perhaps more on the relationships that form. At Takoma Village, a member has dementia, and she continues to live there on her own. Neighbors remind her when it's time to come to group dinners, and she attends occasional activities. She pays for someone to come for a few hours each day to help her, and so far, it's working out. When she had to go to a rehabilitation facility after a fall, Ann visited her and found that the woman's daughter was proactive about putting the pieces together for her mother to stay at Takoma Village as long as possible.

Ann, who is very active in the cohousing movement, began to use a wheelchair when she was in her fifties. That change in her mobility made her appreciate cohousing even more. "It would be so much harder to live independently," she said. "Every ounce of energy I have would be sapped." One neighbor does Ann's weekly grocery shopping and others offer help as needed. Because she is usually at home, she reciprocates by taking in packages that are delivered or letting in repair people for neighbors.

Whether cohousing can delay the need to move to long-term care has not been proven, but many members believe it to be true. "I do feel you can stay longer," said Ann. That said, she would not expect to remain if she were unable to get out of bed in the morning and take care of her own physical needs.

Bob has lived with his wife and daughter at Pleasant Hill Cohousing in Pleasant Hill, California, since 2001, and like Ann Zabaldo he can't imagine living anywhere but cohousing. Pleasant Hill has a wide range of ages, with a large crop of kids and many retirees who act as surrogate aunts and uncles. Bob said he always knew cohousing was a great place to live, but over time he's also come to believe that "it's a great place to die."

He tells the story of Jay, a sixty-year-old member of their community who was diagnosed with colon cancer. From his first appointment with the oncologist, Jay had neighbors accompany him and help him every step of the way. "I was his 'science advisor,'" said Bob, who is a medical writer. "We have a member who's a minister who was his spiritual advisor, and another member was his financial advisor. Jay was single his whole life, no children, and his only close relative lived in Chicago. But he had all of us." Nobody loved cohousing more than Jay did, said Bob, because of the connections.

Jay was given an eighteen-month prognosis, but he lived for three years. Initially, his cohousing family helped him cook meals and get to medical appointments, but it became too much. One of his friends there urged him to hire a patient advocate to take over many of those tasks, which he agreed to do. "That helped a lot," said Bob. "It allowed us in the community to support him without actually having to disrupt our lives every day. This patient advocate did so much for him and became a personal friend of his. It worked out very well."

When it became clear that Jay had not long to live, the community planned a celebration of his life, with a catered dinner in the common house and lots of friends from various parts of his life. "The day we had that dinner is the day he took a turn for the worse," Bob recalls.

He could not attend the dinner, but they brought him home from the hospital to spend his last few days in hospice care. We were all singing a song that we sing as they wheeled him out of the ambulance. For the next three days, every child came by to spend time with him. We all came to sing with him and be with him. It was wonderful. On the morning he died, one of his neighbors, Elaine, went to visit him and started singing show tunes—'We Could Have Danced all Night.' He raised his arms and was dancing—a few hours before he died. I want his death.

CHAPTER 5

Cooperatives
Living Affordably

In the high desert of central Oregon on a crisp October morning, Dick Martin led me on a tour of the Green Pastures Senior Community where he lives. Green Pastures, a housing cooperative of mobile homes, sits on the edge of Redmond, a thriving town of twenty-seven thousand people.

The high desert is on an immense plateau that stretches eastward from the foothills of the Cascades range. Surrounding the town are acres of fields, dried golden in the arid climate, the only swatches of green from acreage still being irrigated before winter sets in.

Green Pastures appears as serene as its name suggests. The community, comprised of fifty-one lots—forty-nine of them with homes—laid out in three adjacent sections, is tidy, with bursts of pink and gold from marigolds, petunias, and chrysanthemums planted near doorsteps. Manufactured homes have come a long way from their roots in trailer parks. The housing type—the preferred name now is mobile or manufactured—is ideal for people with disabilities or who have age-related mobility problems. The homes are a pleasant combination of feeling both roomy and compact, with all the amenities of a traditional (also known as stick-built) ranch-style house.

I've come to Green Pastures to get a feel for what life is like in a homeowner cooperative for people fifty-five and over. Dick Martin led the effort to organize the co-op, and he combines the roles of de facto mayor, maintenance supervisor, cheerleader, and helpful neighbor. He's a tall, confident Westerner, can-do but not blustery. Ramona, his wife of fifty-seven years, is soft-spoken and sweet, and seems equally committed to the cooperative venture.

As we walked through the park, Dick related something of each co-op member's story—the couple in their eighties who are both itinerant preachers; the country music legend; the woman whose pioneering grandfather laid out the streets of nearby Bend; the family who chose to buy two homes in the park, for two generations to live side by side.

Susan, out sweeping her porch on this chilly morning, stops to chat. "I love it here," she said. "It's quiet, peaceful. It's the calmest place I've ever been. My neighbors are nice."

Bob Gibson, a wise-cracking country and western guitar player and songwriter who performed in the old days with Willie, Merle, and Johnny, said he likes it here fine. "We're just a bunch of old guys hanging on by our fingernails," he jokes of his neighbors. "You reach that point in life where you don't want all those burdens, where you don't want all those chores." (He also offers such sage words as, "Don't hang around the senior center. You'll get depressed." and "You can tell where the seniors are—where all the Buicks are parked.")

He and his wife, Carol, also a performer, clear out for Yuma, Arizona, half the year, to get away from the snow, but otherwise plan to stay at Green Pastures. "If you're a senior you cannot find a better deal and a better place to live than a co-op like this," he said. "If you can help your neighbor a little bit or they can help you, what's wrong with that?"

Across the country and a world away, in a canyon of high-rise apartments in Manhattan, similar sentiments are echoed by members of Penn South, an intergenerational housing cooperative of five thousand members living in three thousand apartments in ten huge brick buildings in the Chelsea neighborhood. Stretched across the fence along a parking lot, an immense banner celebrated the co-op's fiftieth anniversary in 2012.

The Penn South members I met said that their cooperative is fundamentally different from a condominium or rental apartments. "A cooperative is affordable and nonprofit and self-governing," as Harriet, a long-time member, explained it. "There should be a lot more places like this."

At first glance, Green Pastures and Penn South seem to have little in common. One is age restricted, the other not. One is rural, the other urban. One is comprised of mobile homes, the other apartments. But they are variations on the cooperative themes of member-owned and democratically run, with a strong sense of community as the foundation. Both are officially considered affordable housing by their respective jurisdictions and qualify for subsidized grants and loans.

Penn South and Green Pastures are among the 6,400 housing cooperatives in the United States made up of 1.2 million dwellings, representing 1 percent of all housing units in the country in 2010. Of that 1.2 million, 425,000 are limited- or zero-equity, meaning they were established to remain affordable, with each member's share of the co-op increasing in value at a modest fixed rate, rather than fluctuating with the market. The other 775,000 units are market rate, with the price of each rising—or falling—with prevailing housing costs.[1] In the case of manufactured home parks, co-op members each own their home, but the cooperative owns the land on which the home sits, ensuring it will not be sold out from under the members.

In addition to manufactured home parks and high-rise apartment buildings, cooperatives can be single-family homes, such as in Village Creek in

Norwalk, Connecticut, whose founders successfully integrated their community in 1949, a time when black and white people were seldom neighbors. In Greenbelt, Maryland, one of the first planned, federally-owned communities in the nation (see next chapter for more on Greenbelt and Penn South), the housing cooperative is made up predominantly of townhouses.

The notion of multiple families dividing a structure and sharing ownership is hardly new. According to one account of the historical roots of cooperatives, records from 2000 BC referred to people owning different floors of a house, for example. One document, "a condominium-type deed written on papyrus dating from 434 BC," described an apartment unit whose owner had the rights of conveyance and title insurance.[2]

In our own country, "More than 1,000 years ago the Pueblo Indians in the southwest carved their apartment-like homes from the side of mountains. They did not know it then, but these native American cliff dwellers could have been considered some of the first developers of residential cooperative housing in the world," the article notes.[3]

In the United States, housing cooperatives, originally called "home clubs," were first built in the nineteenth century in New York City, initially as luxury housing for the well-to-do. But between the two World Wars, co-ops for people of modest means were organized, often by trade unions.[4]

New York led the way in passing laws to encourage cooperative development. In 1926, the state's Limited Dividends Housing Companies Act was passed, in large part to replace dangerous tenements with quality affordable housing. Developers were given incentives to construct low-income, cooperatively-owned apartment housing. According to an account of cooperative housing on Manhattan's Lower East Side, "Private investors were slow in taking on such projects. But the incentives did appeal to others. Civic-minded and progressive men were actively working to remedy the housing situation. The unions in particular were interested not only in improving the working conditions of its [sic] members but also in their general welfare. They were inspired by democratic-socialist ideas and social movements that grew in response to industrialism and the harsh working conditions in factories and sweatshops."[5]

One of the first organizations to embrace cooperative housing for the masses was the Amalgamated Clothing Workers Union, which created the Amalgamated Housing Corporation. Its housing co-ops, including Hillman Houses and East River Housing, still remain.[6]

Penn South has similar roots. It was organized in 1957, with financial and moral support from the International Ladies Garment Workers Union. Each household has one share in the cooperative, entitling members to lifetime residency and one vote in co-op decision making. The city has helped Penn South remain affordable through various property tax-relief measures that have been reaffirmed by the membership and continue today.[7]

Cooperatives are similar to condominiums, in that owners have their own units and share financial responsibility for the common spaces. But they differ legally, financially, and philosophically. In general, co-ops are more explicit about members being part of a whole and in many cases have a stronger sense of community and joint ownership. (That said, the cooperative-condominium differences are muddied by the fact that co-housing communities, discussed in the previous chapter, generally are set up as condominiums, although some are cooperatives.) Cooperatives of all stripes—from the local food co-op to the rural electric cooperative—at least in theory subscribe to seven core principles:

- voluntary and open membership
- democratic member control
- members' economic participation
- autonomy and independence for each co-op
- member education and training
- cooperation among cooperatives
- concern for the wider community

These principles are meant to encourage members to take responsibility for the shared enterprise and to look out for one another.

Aging Cooperatively

Most housing co-ops are multigenerational, like Penn South, but the numbers of senior housing co-ops like Green Pastures are slowly growing. In either case, housing cooperatives can be ideal settings for people as they age. "They get the feeling of the strength of the community behind them; they can feel relaxed as much as possible," said Nat Yalowitz. "People are much more at ease and that contributes to their health and their wellbeing."

A 2001 research report on rural communities that had established senior housing co-ops identified multiple benefits of this type of ownership:

- Financially, people preserve their home equity and enjoy homeowner tax advantages. Older people keep control over their housing and their lives.

- Maintenance, landscaping, housekeeping, and transportation expenses are shared.[8]
- The community is supportive and safe, yet independent and affordable.
- People remain in their own communities as they age and contribute to the social, spiritual, and financial health of their home town.
- Both independence and interdependence are nurtured.[9]

At a 2005 public forum in Washington, DC, "Cooperative Solutions for Seniors," organized by the Cooperative Development Foundation, leaders from around the nation met at the National Press Club to swap stories. One lesson that some may find surprising: "Low-income people (mostly women) in their seventies and eighties can run a large organization and lots of real estate, very successfully," according to Fred Wood, general manager of CSI Support & Development Services.[10]

As gerontologist Gerry Glaser with the nonprofit Ebenezer Center for Aging in Minneapolis said in testimony in 1981 on the advantages of housing cooperatives for older people's wellbeing:

> From a gerontological point of view, the essential benefit of the cooperative is that it provides an economic structure and social framework that fosters self reliance, self control and determination, interdependence and cooperation among the resident members, even among those with severe chronic conditions. As gerontologists we know that these factors contribute directly to continued independent living, successful aging and the enhancement of longer life. It is possible that some of those critical social forces could emerge in a condominium approach, though we are not so sure. Likened to an ocean voyage, in a condominium each of us ties our individual boats together and sets sail. By contrast, with the cooperative, each of us sets sail on the same ship for better or worse. In short, in the cooperative "we are all in it together."[11]

The first senior housing co-op, called 7500 York Cooperative, was completed in Edina, Minnesota, in 1978. Made up of 338 apartments, the community is thriving. Since then one hundred senior housing co-ops have been built, mostly in Minnesota and other upper Midwestern states, with a smattering elsewhere.[12]

One in Bellevue, Washington, is Silver Glen Cooperative. Betty Ann moved there from Milwaukee, after her husband died. In Wisconsin, she was living alone on a lake, far from her children, two of whom lived on the East Coast and two on the West. Her daughter suggested she check out Silver Glen.

"The word 'co-op' gave me reassurance," said Betty Ann. "I'm familiar with co-ops. I lived in North Dakota and I realized the farmer's union was a co-op and what a wonderful thing it was for farmers." When her daughter called to say Silver Glen had an opening, Betty Ann made her move. "I was eighty-five at the time," she said. "I knew I wasn't going to get any younger."

What she found was a vibrant community where people seem to live long and well. "People are living to be so old here," she said. "I think it's because you are so involved. You're taking care of yourself, and you're so involved in the community, and I think it's what keeps people going."

Not that her neighbors don't face challenges. In fact, she said, "Many are not well at all, but they love the spirit of independence. For me, it's that spirit that keeps people going here." Betty Ann is on the leadership team, helping with finances. Like many communities, the co-op has a wellness committee, a fitness room, and the usual bridge clubs. Much of the landscaping and maintenance is done by co-op members who volunteer. "Some can hardly walk, but they still go out with a spade and do what they can," said Betty Ann. "We do a lot ourselves. I find it quite an exciting place."

Senior housing co-ops, like senior cohousing, do not provide continuing care, such as assisted living or skilled nursing. (An exception is 7500 York, which in 2011 opened an adjoining building that offers assisted living, memory care, and apartments for rehabilitation.) Yet some believe that the relationships that people form may allow them to stay in their own homes longer than they might otherwise, without formal assistance. No promises are made to those moving in, but supportive relationships evolve naturally through everyday life in the community. At Silver Glen, one woman who died of cancer received a tremendous amount of help from the community, in addition to paid in-home care. "It was the people here in our building that allowed her to die here," said Betty Ann. "They'd come in during the night. It's quite beautiful."

Although she understands the appeal of living in a multigenerational community, Betty Ann said she enjoys living just with her peers. "At eighty-five, I had to face it, I was a senior," she said with a laugh. "I just turned ninety. This is where I belong. There is the downside that one does face death more. I feel here, even though we're getting older and people are dying, there's an optimism about each day."

Being comfortable with the yin and yang of enjoying life even as death grows nearer seems to be a gift that some elders embrace. Reflecting on how it felt to turn ninety, Betty Ann said, "It was a strange feeling. On the one side, there was 'Roll out the barrel,' and the other side, 'Take my hand, precious Lord, take my hand.'"

Like many organizations that are age-restricted, whether traditional retirement communities, cohousing, or cooperatives, Silver Glen struggles to attract the younger end of the fifty-five-and-over spectrum. Increasingly, people who move there are in their eighties or even nineties.

Green Pastures seems to be somewhat more successful at attracting "younger" people. When I visited, the newest co-op member was in his fifties. The lure of living in an inexpensive manufactured housing park may be enough to overcome any qualms baby boomers might have about moving to a seniors community. "Our hope is that people who will buy here are in their sixties," said Dick Martin. "They'll stay longer and volunteer more."

Rural Cooperative Living

Paul Bradley, founding president of ROC USA (for Resident-Owned Communities), is a national leader in promoting conversion of privately-owned mobile home parks to cooperatives. People outside of rural areas, who have been known to stigmatize residents of these communities as "trailer trash," likely do not realize the important role played by mobile or manufactured homes in providing affordable housing. In all, there are roughly forty-eight thousand mobile home parks nationally. One in four low-income homeowners in rural communities lives in a mobile home, representing the largest source of unsubsidized low-income housing in the nation.[13] Only a small percentage of the parks have organized cooperatives; most are privately owned. The homeowners who live in private parks are constantly at risk that the land on which they live will be sold out from under them, leading to what Bradley calls "ugly surprises."

"Community closure is a horrible experience, a horrible surprise for any homeowner," he said. "When people buy a home, they buy it believing it's a secure place to live out their lives. And unless you have control of the land beneath your home, you don't enjoy that long-term security."

The way to get that security, he continued, is through a resident-owned housing cooperative. "When all the stars align, most homeowners are in favor of that," he said. "Our job is to help make the stars align, arranging the resources to purchase their communities and providing the opportunity and wherewithal to do that."

New Hampshire leads the way in mobile home cooperatives, with more than one hundred parks, made up of nearly 5,700 homeowners, converting from private to resident ownership from 1984 to 2013.

Lois Parris, president of Lakes Region Mobile Home Park Cooperative in

Belmont, New Hampshire, was a convert. When their park went on the market in 2000, the residents were not prepared to buy it. "We were not at that time able to get the funding," she recalled. "We kept filing with the state and praying we'd get a second chance."

Their prayers were answered, thanks to help from the New Hampshire Community Loan Fund. Not only did the Fund help with financing, said Lois, but the Fund's staff are there for the long haul to help homeowners learn to be effective cooperative owners. "Part of it is the training that's involved," she said. "You don't just buy the community and walk away. It requires constant training. [The Community Loan Fund] is always there. They keep track of you. You always have a place to go. There's training for board members. It's more than just saying 'here, buy the park and good luck.'"

Most of these co-ops are for people of all ages. "I do not want to live in a fifty-five-and-over park," said Lois. "I think it's good medicine for us as we get older to have families and the community feeling. I have my sister who lives across the street from me. We can help each other."

Local nonprofits in Oregon were also pivotal to members of Green Pastures becoming a cooperative. When the Martins arrived in 2006, they intended it to be their last move. The late park owner at that time was a somewhat eccentric woman named Alice Teater. According to Dick's written account of the park:

> Alice was a lover of animals, especially horses. She had a big corral
> built next to her home, where she could see the horses from her house.
> Nevertheless, she restricted the animals allowed in the Park. Of course, no
> mobile home owners and renters were allowed to have horses. And, there
> would be a very limited number of cats and dogs. Alice also refused to have
> any trees or limbs removed from the many trees in the Park. If a tree limb
> began to hang, the limb would be strapped and tied up to a higher limb,
> but it would not be removed.

Before Alice Teater died in 2003, she had bequeathed the entire parcel of land to two local humane societies. They in turn needed cash and decided to sell it. Suddenly, residents were at risk of being forced to move.

In March 2008, Dick and Ramona returned home from shopping to find a letter stuck in their door from the Northwest Cooperative Development Center, inviting park residents to a meeting at the Redmond Senior Center to learn about forming a cooperative. Cohosting the gathering was the nonprofit Community and Shelter Assistance Corporation of Oregon (CASA).

Park residents turned out for the initial meeting and unanimously expressed interest in learning more about how they might form a cooperative. The concept lit a fire under Dick. As he recalled, "Ramona lost me for a year and a half." He composed a detailed letter explaining to his neighbors why a cooperative would be in their best interest. He went door to door, delivering the letter and answering questions.

Dick had never been involved with a cooperative before, but he had a lifetime of leadership and problem-solving under his belt. As a young man, he had begun his career sweeping floors at a heavy equipment shop in Springfield, Oregon, and soon learned to be a welder, then a mechanic. He did a stint with GE, supervising machining projects from Alaska to Nevada. He spent the last eighteen years before his retirement as an operations supervisor, back in the Springfield shop where he'd gotten his start.

When he and Ramona first retired in 2000, they wintered in Yuma, then grew adventurous and lived year-round at their home in the high Cascades. Although the setting was idyllic, the Martins began thinking it was too remote and unrealistic for the long haul. They moved to Redmond to be near their daughter and grandkids, and bought a manufactured home in Green Pastures.

Overnight, with the threat of the land being sold, the secure future they had envisioned was at risk. Park residents learned that an appraiser had determined that the new owners would likely get more money by selling the property to a developer to build single-family homes than by preserving it as a manufactured housing park. If this transpired, it could cost each family as much as $14,000 just to move their homes. Oregon law mandated they be given 365 days to move, and that the new owners compensate them $7000 of the costs. "Fortunately, the State of Oregon also passed the 'Preserving Affordable Housing Act' which became our salvation," Dick wrote.

According to Oregon law, the park qualifies as affordable housing since at least 60 percent of households earn 80 percent or less of the area median income—roughly less than $42,000 in 2012.

Also working in residents' favor was Alice Teater's expressed wish that any future sale be to someone who wanted to preserve the property as a manufactured home park.

Dick and Ramona and seven other residents organized a steering committee and were guided by the Northwest Center and CASA in the intricacies of financing and legalities. At each juncture where a decision had to be made, the residents of Green Pastures voted unanimously to take the next step in forming a cooperative.

In August 2008 at a pivotal meeting called to vote on whether to proceed formally with organizing a cooperative and buying the park, Ramona and another volunteer sat at tables while park residents lined up. Homeowners each had to put down $500 to indicate their intention to join the co-op. Before the meeting even started, 100 percent of the residents had stood in line and officially indicated their intent to join the fledgling cooperative. "Neither CASA of Oregon nor NW Cooperative Development Center could believe our success. This meeting was designed to encourage everyone to sign up. I think they were wondering why we were having the meeting. The signup had been completed. Oh well, we all got free coffee and cookies," Dick wrote.[14]

As Dick relates this story, it's clear that the act of organizing such an ambitious undertaking, which involved securing a $1.4 million loan and having responsibility for the park, all served to bring the residents closer together. "Since we formed this cooperative, people are getting to know each other," Dick told me. "Before this, when the trust owned this park and we paid rent, it was surprising how few people knew each other. It's a good community, and everybody gets along real well."

As far as house and community design, Green Pastures seems ideal for people as they age. The homes are compact and one-level and can also be made more accessible with wheelchair ramps and other accommodations. Crime is almost unheard of—the worst thing that has happened was a statue being swiped out of someone's yard. The park has high quality medical facilities and shopping just minutes away. "For a senior, it's a pretty handy place to live," Dick said.

The community lacks a meeting space for social gatherings so they rent the local senior center. An informal support network assists members, several of whom are in their nineties. "A lady here, her husband passed away," said Dick. "Then she had a stroke, and they took her driver's license away from her. She had two neighbors right away chauffeuring her around. They jumped in and almost started arguing about who got to chauffeur." Dick and Ramona often help some of the older women with rides, and Dick mows lawns for four widows.

The co-op keeps rules to a minimum. Dogs and cats (on leash) are welcome now, unlike when Alice Teater ruled the roost. One cat owner is Phyllis, the community's oldest member at ninety-four and the sister of Alice Teater. As I was talking to the Martins in their living room, Phyllis knocked on the door. She needed help getting her cat, Sophie, out of its crate—it was hard for Phyllis to crouch down and lean into the crate to grab Sophie. Sophie came there by way of Phyllis's daughter, supposedly as a favor to the daughter. "You know what that means," said Phyllis. "She thinks I need a cat."

Phyllis is a diminutive woman with deep roots in central Oregon. "This was my sister's horse ranch," she said. "I never dreamed I'd be living here. The nicest thing is the people."

Phyllis had worked for the Red Cross in Europe and lived in Alaska. Her ancestors were leading pioneers in nearby Bend. Her grandfather engineered the irrigation systems, and laid out the streets there in 1900. Phyllis herself was recently crowned Queen of the Deschutes Pioneers (Deschutes is the name of the river and the county).

She invites us to stroll over to her house. After Dick retrieves Sophie from her crate, we go inside. Phyllis's home seems large—more than 1,200 square feet, with three bedrooms and a living room big enough for a piano and a small organ. She used to play piano and accordion to entertain folks at senior centers.

The backyard has a peach tree laden with fruit. Ramona said Phyllis always wants to return any favors. When Dick does a home repair or mows her lawn, she'll appear at the Martins with a fresh peach or even a few potatoes she's bought. She shares her newspaper with another neighbor and every day walks over and delivers it to the woman.

Phyllis likes the concept of a cooperative. "People can have their own rules," she said. "The people here know what to do."

I ask if she hopes to remain here, and she does. "Of course I could die at any time," she said matter-of-factly. Dick points out she's been saying that as long as he's known her. She smiles.

The cooperative seems to have created a community that serves its members in many ways. For one, it's hard to imagine a more affordable way to be a homeowner. In addition to the $500 membership fee (which is refunded if you move), members pay $350 a month to the cooperative to cover property taxes, a rainy-day fund, community landscaping, and other shared expenses. The price of the homes themselves varies considerably, depending on the age, size, and amenities. One recently-purchased home in fine condition sold for $17,000.

But perhaps as importantly, a cooperative, by its nature, gives members a sense of purpose, as they must manage the property and the organization in a way that benefits everyone. The close proximity of neighbors encourages people to help one another, even if they can't drive or if they have physical or cognitive challenges.

It must feel really satisfying to have organized the cooperative, I said to Dick. "I guess I just feel a moral obligation to assist in the leadership of our community," he said. "Not only a moral obligation, but a real feeling of satisfaction. Sometimes I feel like I'm to a big degree the protector of some of the folks in our community. I will probably continue this role as long as I can."

CHAPTER 6

NORCs
Retiring Naturally

In the mid-1980s, Nat Yalowitz looked around and realized that his beloved community, Penn South Cooperative, was growing old. Some 70 percent of co-op members were over sixty. Like Nat and his wife, many had moved to the co-op in the 1960s to raise their families and live affordably in Manhattan. Although Nat didn't know the term at the time, what he had identified at Penn South was a Naturally Occurring Retirement Community (NORC), a neighborhood, apartment complex, or town with a high concentration of older people.

It didn't take much imagination for Nat to realize that his neighbors might soon be facing age-related challenges that could threaten the stability and vitality of the community. A social worker himself, Nat observed the other co-op members through the lens not only of a friend and neighbor but of a professional. He observed that for many people who retired, the ground shifted under them as they discovered that the routines, purpose, and companions of the workplace were not easy to replace.

"Things can become somewhat disorganized for some people," he wrote later.

> They begin to feel off balance and without a plan or a network of people they can relate to on a regular basis. Spousal tension at home can begin to take place and some beginning loss of identity can result. Workers . . . with limited income found themselves somewhat hard pressed; some began to show signs of feeling depressed, anxious, and lonely, and some seemed to lack any support network while others seemed to lack adequate medical care. There was a sense of lack of structure and of things coming apart.[1]

Nat is not a handwringer. Like Dick Martin of Green Pastures, Nat is a problem solver. With the blessing of the Board of Directors, he conducted a survey of the co-op to learn more about members' problems and needs. That led to the co-op contributing $8,000 in seed money for a part-time social worker from a nearby social service nonprofit to serve Penn South's older members.

Nat's vision was not limited to social work, though. For one, he wanted to ensure that the members maintained control of the organization and were not made to feel like passive recipients of help. He began to plan a holistic and comprehensive set of services and programs to support co-op members who wanted to stay rooted in their community. Rather than a scattershot approach, where people have to find and negotiate a myriad of programs—transportation, cultural, educational, social, home improvement, wellness, financial, and so on—Penn South would bring all these and more to the community and give members a one-stop way to connect. In 1986, Penn South created the first comprehensive Naturally Occurring Retirement Community supportive services program (NORC-SSP), now a model for the nation.

The term "NORC" was introduced in a 1986 article by Michael Hunt, a professor of design at University of Wisconsin–Madison, and his wife Gail Gunter-Hunt, a social worker with the Veteran's Hospital. The Hunts identified what they believed was the most common form of retirement community in the nation: not a planned one, but one that evolved in an area where a significant number of people were aging in place. They meant a majority, but today NORCs refer to communities with a concentration of older people, even if it is far less than half the population. Typically a NORC is comprised of people who have lived in their homes for decades, never leaving after raising their families. Less frequently, they include people who have migrated there to retire. But unlike a traditional planned retirement community, a NORC exists with no thought having been given to the changing needs of older residents. NORCs "are also of interest because older people are attracted to them naturally, without formal advertising, even though the housing was not designed or planned for older people," the Hunts wrote.[2]

For these "natural" retirement communities to serve older people well, the Hunts found, key services need to be nearby, ideally within one-half mile. Such services include a grocery, drugstore, bank, variety store, department store, post office, doctor's office, dry cleaners, library, churches (and other houses of worship), and restaurants. "These may be more important than the house itself," they wrote, concluding, a "NORC allows older people to benefit from a supportive neighborhood and frequent contact with age peers, while still living independently in an age-integrated neighborhood."[3]

Today the term NORC has come to mean something more than just a demographic description. Around the country, places like Penn South have begun to realize that they can be proactive about identifying and meeting the needs of their older populations by creating NORC-SSPs. That unwieldy acronym has been conflated, and NORC-SSPs are often referred to simply as NORCs. Although NORCs vary considerably in size and services, they generally embrace a philosophy of empowerment and a commitment to assisting people in remaining vital and in charge of their lives.

This contrasts with the typical social-service model. "Seniors will object to being considered a 'case' managed by a professional as though they have stopped being thoughtful and responsible for their own lives," Yalowitz wrote. "Instead, we call this helping process care coordination."[4]

Amy Chalfy, who supervises services offered by the Jewish Association Serving the Aged (JASA) at Penn South, has worked with older people in a variety of settings for decades. She's never seen anything like Penn South. "In other communities, older people are much more segregated," she said. "With the NORC program people are able to contribute and to be involved, and that strengthens the whole community. It took a lot of vision to make this happen. This is a different ball game. As a model, it's tremendous."

Unlike Villages, which are typically membership-based, NORCs offer services to all older people (and sometimes people of all ages with disabilities as well) in a given locale. NORCs usually offer more services than Villages and do so by partnering with agencies already working in the community, rather than reinventing the wheel. NORCs were given a boost following the 2005 White House Conference on Aging, which directed money to underserved elders aging in place.[5] Researchers have been studying the model, and Congress funded some fifty pilot projects in twenty-six states between 2002 and 2010, in hopes of both meeting people's desire to remain in their homes and saving money by preventing or delaying institutional long-term care.[6] A small federal Community Innovations for Aging in Place program also supports NORC-type projects.[7]

By the mid-1990s, other housing cooperatives in New York had followed Penn South's lead and established NORCs, including Co-op City in the Bronx, the largest housing co-op in the country with more than fifteen thousand apartments. The programs have been supported by a mix of foundation grants; public funds; contributions, both financial and in-kind from the housing co-ops themselves; and modest fees paid by members for classes or activities. By 1997 Nat was receiving so many inquiries he created another entity, the NORC Supportive Services Center, Inc., to advise emerging NORCs around the country. They have since guided a couple dozen organizations and agencies, mostly in New York, but also in Illinois, Michigan, and Maryland.

Nationally, more than eighty NORC-SSP programs in twenty-five states are part of the National NORCs Aging in Place Initiative organized by The Jewish Federations of North America, the leader in the world of NORCs.[8]

୧୨

I was eager to visit Penn South and one hot summer day I boarded a Megabus from Washington and headed up to New York. I met Nat in Manhattan's Chelsea neighborhood, a pleasant mix of apartment buildings, restaurants, and shops. Penn South is a behemoth: a complex of huge brick buildings, housing as many as five thousand people in nearly three thousand apartments. Nat met me outside and led me through a warren of rooms in the bowels of one of the buildings. One room had a sign cautioning "Meditation in Progress—Do Not Disturb." Another was a sculpture studio. Others were used as offices, bustling with staff who are there to serve the older co-op members through the Penn South Program for Seniors (PSPS).

We ended up sitting around a small table in a windowless office, part of the space donated by the housing co-op to PSPS. Nat had invited a few of the co-op members—Sonia, Harriet, and Jason—to fill me in on the expansive program that is the fruit of Nat's vision. They are active participants as well as leaders through service on the PSPS board.

Sonia, eighty-five, a "newcomer," moved to the co-op only a decade ago. When her husband was alive, they were not eligible to live at Penn South because their income was too high. "I was in a really good marriage, and he up and died on me," she said. "I was grieving. I was a wreck."

She decided to shake the dice and apply for an apartment in the co-op. When she got the call that one was available, she did not hesitate. "I'm really happy," she said. "It's the right apartment and the right place. I really feel I'm maintaining my quality of life."

At Penn South, I learned, people have plenty of opportunity to develop leadership, to be engaged with the world beyond its walls, and to live with purpose and pleasure. As Nat put it, "If it can't be fun, I'm not interested."

Like Nat, Harriet arrived fifty years ago and raised her kids there. "It was a great place to live when I was much younger, and it was always a community where people were helpful," she said. "I felt fortunate to live here. It became an enriching community—there were playgroups for the children. The fact that when we age we have our friends around us, it makes life better."

The natural interaction among the generations that is part of any strongly bonded community, whether it's a congregation or a small town, is part of everyday life here—partly spontaneous, partly planned. "In our building," said Sonia, "[older] people sit on benches in the lobby. The little ones come by for their pat."

Nat trumped her: "In my building they come for a hug."

Besides these casual encounters, PSPS has unusually rich intergenerational offerings. Too often at retirement communities or nursing homes, "intergenerational" means children or teens troop through at holidays and perform to an audience of passive old people. While this may be better than no contact at all, it's a poor substitute for a genuine exchange. Penn South offers many such opportunities. The co-op holds an annual arts festival for all age groups that includes musical performances, singing, and poetry reading. One much beloved art teacher was still volunteering when he was ninety-nine. Children and elders work together on a community garden and on quilting—putting older people in their traditional role of teacher, rather than mere recipient.

Beyond kids who live at the co-op, Penn South has many programs involving students of all ages from the wider community. Sonia shared one of many examples. "I was in an intergenerational program with a high school fashion and design class. We met one-on-one or in small groups. The students really wanted to know about my life. Then they did an art project—a shadow outline of your face and decorated it." Other co-op members participate in an arts program with children from the public elementary school across the street. In an oral history partnership with the City University of New York Masters Applied Theater program, students interviewed co-op members, then dramatized their life stories. "It's amazing, seeing how much joy and understanding it brings to both sides," said Nat.

Jason, a slender man with longish hair, said he's grateful for the senior services program. "It's been sustaining to me to have classes here," he said. "One was called Talking Pictures. Two guys came from the School of Visual Arts. We have comedy improv and drama. We have shows. It's given me an opportunity to do something very meaningful to me. Another woman who lost her husband has used it as a bulwark."

Another unusual collaboration took place between older co-op members and students at the nearby campus of the Fashion Institute of Technology. As Nat wrote:

> Several years ago, a professor there approached the NORC program with the idea that his interior design class could work closely with a group of seniors to redesign their homes at no cost. . . . Many seniors were interested in this even after learning that a lot of work would be involved on their part. They were not phased one bit by this and the project was

started. . . . Everyone was astonished at the tremendous enthusiasm on the part of the students and seniors. These young students gave seniors a sense that their ideas would be listened to and the seniors grew giddy from the entire process. These seniors were absolutely enthralled by what had taken place in terms of redesigning their homes following many of their own ideas and resulting in more comfortable, beautiful, safe, inviting and economically doable home projects.[9]

New York and other cities can be exceptional places to grow old, in part due to good public transportation and an endless array of cultural resources. At Penn South, for example, musicians from Carnegie Hall come to perform. "It's like a salon," said Nat. "They are able to have a wonderful exchange with the audience—about art history, music history."

Although such programs sounded appealing to me, PSPS has trouble attracting co-op members who are my age—a lament I was to hear at many other places I visited. We discussed why this might be. The group wondered if having the word "senior" in the program's name is off-putting.

Nat blamed it partly on ageism.

Harriet thought it was denial, on the part of people of all ages. "People won't use canes and walkers," she said of her peers. "We all have preconceived notions of being old. We all assume you don't grow, or if you do, you don't have talent. The wonderful thing about this group is you can do things you never dreamed you could do—you discover aspects of your life that you never dreamed of. One woman in my drama group had never acted before—she loves it."

Added Jason, "It's a place for people coming out." By that he did not mean coming out of the closet, but out of their ruts of lifelong routines and identities and finding undiscovered talents.

"We've had people who have written poetry which we've published," said Nat. "We've had people who have never been leaders who are now activists, people who never acted who have been in commercial films."

"It's supportive and enhancing," agreed Sonia.

It's this spirit of growth, of surprise, of living fully that lured Harriet into becoming active in the seniors program. "It never occurred to me—I was in my seventies—that this organization would have anything to offer me," she laughed. In other words, the seniors program was for old people, for people who needed help, not for folks like Harriet.

The first thing that drew her in was the computer class—one of thirty educational classes PSPS offers. She was embarrassed that her grandson knew more than she did about computers. Then came art history. "I made new friends," she said. "If someone doesn't see me in class, they call me. It's been a wonderful experience for me. It's a form of blossoming."

I asked if there's something in the water at Penn South—the folks I met are "old" by most standards—in their late seventies to mid-eighties—but they are among the most vital and growing of anyone I've met, of any age. The contrast between the popular image of a traditional retirement community—daily doses of card games and golf—is striking. Nat was eighty-three and was hoping to groom younger leaders to step up.

It seems to demonstrate what some researchers theorize and what *The Blue Zones* project that looked at centenarians found: old age as a period of decline may be a social construct, just as Penn South's culture of generativity and fun is a social construct, but one more life-enhancing than we've been led to believe was possible for older people.

Although this small group wanted to focus on the social, educational, and cultural experiences they'd had, those are only a part of what the NORC offers. I also talked with Elaine Rosen and Chris Diaz who help provide care coordination for a hundred fifty members. With 55 percent of the co-op's members over sixty, they are kept busy, receiving referrals almost daily for everything from someone falling, to becoming disoriented, to being discharged from the hospital.

"Our goal is to keep people in their home safely and for them to stay active in the community," said Elaine. She credits Nat for spearheading the program.

"When we started doing it, it was practical, not revolutionary," he said modestly.

Chris jumped in: "But it's really innovative."

"With a huge impact," added Elaine.

Aging in place, done right, requires an intense amount of coordination, they explain. Often, people who could use some help refuse to ask for it. In addition, well-meaning relatives worry that it's time for their loved ones to move to assisted living or even a nursing home. This may lead elders to conceal emerging problems.

Although they listen to family concerns, Elaine and Chris represent the older people themselves, and they support them if their wish is to remain at Penn South. People with dementia pose the biggest challenge, they said.

Their team includes psychiatrists and psychotherapists who come to Penn South, along with other professionals who provide on-site service. The falls-prevention team, made up of a social worker, a nurse, and a co-op maintenance employee, proactively checks apartments for safety, including ensuring proper lighting. At the same time, people are encouraged to participate in the many exercise classes available. PSPS consulted with medical experts to develop their falls-prevention program, which has been recognized by the state for its results. Nurses also monitor blood pressure and help people manage chronic conditions.

Another program called PS-HOPS (Penn South Home Organized Personal Services) takes advantage of members' shared purchasing power to form a buyers co-op for products and services, including discounted glasses, hearing aids, home health aides, dental care, over-the- counter medications, and other costly items not covered by most insurance plans.

I asked Nat if there's any way to measure the success of the NORC. "Here's the scoop," he said. "Before, when seniors became fragile, they'd go to a hospital—ambulances were here all the time. Some would never come back. Today, those same people stay here. They don't go to a nursing home. There's a tremendous saving of funds. We know a lot of people remain here. We know that every year we've prevented eight to ten people from going to a nursing home." With savings to Medicaid of roughly $80,000 a year by avoiding nursing home placement, Nat estimates as much as $800,000 a year in tax dollars saved—far more than the public gives Penn South in grants.[10] In addition, he said, they are able to prevent many hospitalizations.

Social worker Elaine Rosen adds, "As far as remaining, people stay in their own homes as long as they get the services they need. And we give them the motivation they need."

In 2000 a report of all NORCs in New York State found their service programs "helped forestall 653 hospital stays and 404 nursing home placements."[11] The report found that NORCs' service programs reach "the oldest, frailest and most isolated residents" of their communities. More than one third of these residents had no one to call upon for help, and a similar number needed help with three or more "activities of daily living," such as bathing and dressing—in other words, the type of people whom you'd find in any nursing home.[12] The fact that these elders can remain in their own homes suggests that NORCs may have successfully expanded what is possible through aging in place.

❧

Later that day, Nat took me to a Greek diner in the neighborhood. Joining us was Amy Chalfy of JASA. As I chowed down on a Reuben sandwich, Amy and Nat talked about the significance of what Penn South has accomplished.

"The problem with traditional senior services is you're seen as a recipient," said Amy. "The NORC recognizes people's strengths." She confirmed Nat's belief that Penn South's efforts have kept their members out of assisted living or nursing homes. "The emphasis on reducing isolation is so important. I believe isolation is linked to cognitive and physical decline.

"Penn South is really a remarkable example of what can be done and the partnership that can be created," she continued. "The program promotes the engagement that goes on, and it's a snowball effect."

It goes way beyond offering rides to people or making it easy to get their blood pressure checked. "I think it goes quite deep," said Nat. "I know a lot about their lives."

After lunch, Nat led me on a tour of the area surrounding Penn South. Early on, the co-op wisely bought much of the surrounding property and now leases it to businesses that members want nearby. He pointed out why urban living is ideal for people as they grow old. Within an easy walk from the apartments there's a large supermarket, a tennis court, restaurants, a dry cleaner, and doctor and dentist offices. Beth Israel Hospital rents space from Penn South for a large clinic that serves co-op members. There's even an experimental theater.

Nat is constantly looking for ways to improve and strengthen the apartments' infrastructure. The original windows, for example, were inexpensive and of poor quality; they have all been replaced to improve energy efficiency and help with noise abatement. Amazingly, the co-op even built a cogeneration power plant on its property. "We dumped Con-Ed [Con Edison, the power company] and we're saving $1 million a year in electricity," Nat said proudly. Now they're in the midst of a $100 million project to upgrade the heating, ventilation, and air-conditioning (HVAC) systems in all the buildings.

Although a NORC certainly does not have to be a cooperative, Nat and his co-op peers say that NORCs and co-ops are a natural fit. As Sonia said, "The theme is service. With the co-op you have a sense you're responsible and you care about it. I feel responsible and I have a say."

A Suburban NORC

Most NORCs are likely not as comprehensive as Penn South's, but they still can play a valuable role in supporting people's desire to remain in their own homes and in providing friendship, learning opportunities, and social services. In Rockville, Maryland, social worker Beth Shapiro serves people who want to age in place and who live near each other in older neighborhoods and high-rise apartment buildings in Montgomery County. Through a program called Coming of Age in Maryland, Beth organizes monthly tours, lunch outings to restaurants, and along the way gives mini-counseling sessions and advice. Her list includes 1,200 elders who live in a part of the county with a roughly 20 to 25 percent older population. A recent month's activities included a trip to the National Museum of Women in the Arts and lunch at the café; tickets to see *My Fair Lady* at Arena Stage, a highly regarded Washington, DC, theater; and a day at the Jewish senior center that included exercise, "Table Talk with Beth," lunch, and entertainment by a virtuoso Russian violinist.

"I'll talk to the older adults on the bus," Beth said of the field trips she organizes. "The people know me. If you need to talk to me about a recent fall, about an adult child issue, about where you live, come talk to me. Someone will say, 'Can I talk to you when we get to the museum?' And I'll find a bench for five minutes. If it gets to be a mental health topic, I'll make the referral to another agency for counseling. A professional friendship is what I like to call it."

One small-scale 2010 study suggests there may be benefits from living in a NORC. Researchers compared participants in the nonprofit Community Partners (CP), another NORC social service program in Montgomery County, with their counterparts who chose not to participate. (The latter group was found to be somewhat younger, more male, wealthier, and more highly educated.) Community Partners focused on providing recreational opportunities, transportation, and social work services. The study surveyed residents of six apartment buildings, fifty-eight of whom joined CP and seventy who did not. Of the small number of CP participants who responded to a follow-up survey, more than half said they felt more a part of their building's community, 70 percent said the program had improved their social life, and 88 percent said they would recommend CP to their neighbors. A few said without the program they might have to move, presumably to assisted living or with family. Two-thirds reported they got out of the house more since joining, and nearly that many said they felt happier. A majority felt less isolated after becoming members of CP.

A 2006 national survey conducted by United Jewish Communities of 461 people living in twenty-four NORCs found similar results, with strong majorities of those who participated in NORC programs reporting that they talked to more people, joined in activities or events more than they used to, got out more than before, and knew about and used more community services. Nearly half volunteered more, and nearly three-quarters said they felt healthier. Nearly 90 percent believed they were more likely to remain in the community as a result of the NORC program.[13]

Beth Shapiro is convinced her program helps people stay put. But it's not always simple. She shared the complexities that can arise. "Mrs. Smith," who is in her nineties and walks very slowly, left a message for Beth, saying she wanted to sign up for an upcoming museum trip. Because of Mrs. Smith's mobility problems, Beth didn't think the group could accommodate her. "I had to call Mrs. Smith and explain we weren't totally comfortable, and I got an earful. She put me in my place. She said, 'This is my only way to get out, I can't get to a museum. I'll be damned if you tell me that I can't go, I'm fighting for my life here,'" Beth said. "That's autonomy."

Beth agreed that Mrs. Smith could come, but she said it was hard for her to judge if the older woman could safely get around. Moreover, Beth did not want the whole group to have to walk at Mrs. Smith's pace. Her plan was to find another group at the museum with whom Mrs. Smith could tag along, and Beth would walk with her part of the time, to do an informal assessment. "She's been with us nine years. She's aged in place with our program as have several others. I'll check on how Mrs. Smith is doing and make an assessment as best I can. I don't know what I'll do with that assessment if it's not a good one," she admitted.

As with most NORCs, Coming of Age partners with other agencies to provide a fuller range of services. "We have a mental health partner, a recreation partner, a home health partner, and a bus partner," she said. Beth believes transportation is one of the biggest hurdles for older people: "Not the dementia or frailty. It's all about transportation and getting these folks to the destinations to keep them vital and healthy and engaged with the community."

A New Deal NORC

A different kind of housing co-op with a successful NORC is in Greenbelt, Maryland, just outside Washington, DC. While few of us are likely to live in a high-rise co-op in Manhattan, Greenbelt's experience could be adapted by any municipality with a critical mass of elders and a strong sense of community.

The town has an unusual history as the first federally owned planned community in the nation, founded in 1937. Greenbelt was viewed as a social experiment, created both to provide affordable housing to low-income people and to foster a sense of community. Some 5,700 people applied for the original 885 homes. Those who met income guidelines and professed a strong willingness to participate in community life were chosen. The town's physical layout fosters neighborliness and civic participation.

In the 1950s it converted from federal ownership to a cooperative housing community, and today the whole town is a National Historic Landmark. People take pride in their close-knit progressive culture. The high school is named for Eleanor Roosevelt, and one of Greenbelt's only eating establishments is the New Deal Café. From its inception, Greenbelt's population was a healthy mix of blue-collar workers and professionals, many of whom work at the nearby University of Maryland.

I had often gone to Greenbelt to visit good friends, but never before with an eye for seeing what it's like to grow older there. I asked a sixty-something couple from my congregation if they'd give me an insider's tour. Lola and Steve Skolnik are deeply rooted in Greenbelt, having moved there in 1977. They raised their three children there, and all three have moved back to live within one mile of their parents. Three generations of Skolniks now live in Greenbelt, and some of Lola and Steve's grandchildren attend the same co-op nursery that their own kids went to. "We are not at all unique in that," said Lola, of the deep roots families put down.

On a walking tour, she and Steve point out how the town was designed to nurture community. The homes are grouped in what are called "superblocks," with a system of walking paths that allow people to get to the town center without crossing a major street, making it safe for young and old alike. Underpasses offer additional safe walking beneath the busier streets. The town center, with the municipal building, community center, ball fields, and shops, is built in the middle of a crescent-shaped natural ridge surrounded by the main streets.

Today you won't find fast food joints in old Greenbelt, but you will be able to enjoy a nonprofit Art Deco movie theater, a cooperative bank, a cooperative supermarket, a credit union, and a community playhouse.

"Since we've retired, there's so much to do we don't leave Greenbelt," said Lola. Formerly the director of a senior center, Lola is now devoting her time to pottery, taking advantage of the ceramics studios and kiln in the community center. The center is in the original school and still retains some classrooms with charming wooden cubbies tucked in the walls. It has an impressive offering of classes as well as space for artists-in-residence and for activities for all ages. One room is devoted to costumes for the community theater. In another, women artists were hard at work on their pottery. There are three kilns, a room with a potter's wheel, and another room for those who shape clay by hand. There's a dark room (Steve thinks he may be the only person who uses it in this digital age) and a local-access cable television studio. There's also a large dance studio where Lola takes yoga classes. In a senior lounge, women were knitting, and in the senior game room, a dozen elders were playing bridge.

A chalkboard in the hall listed some twenty activities scheduled for that day alone such as weight watchers, sewing for charity, pre-ballet, a widowed persons support group, and an exercise program called Ageless Grace. Lola said fifty people regularly show up at the gymnasium for the senior fitness class.

The community center is also home to intergenerational activities. Kids who attend the summer camp, for example, put on a circus to which the whole town is invited. On Labor Day a town festival draws thousands each year.

Beyond the community center are indoor and outdoor swimming pools, a youth center, a skateboard park, three baseball fields, tennis courts, and fields for football and soccer. The former bowling alley houses the community theater space. There's also a small lake, dug by hand as part of a Works Progress Administration program in the 1930s.

Lola and Steve both feel that one reason Greenbelt is successful is that so many residents volunteer. Lola has served on the board of the Parks and Recreation Department for thirty years, initially to advocate for people with disabilities. Steve serves on the Board of Appeals, dealing with zoning issues.

"When you see people investing in their community, it makes you want to jump in," said Lola.

They also take advantage of a Prince George's Community College program called SAGE, for Seasoned Adults Growing Educationally. For $50 per semester, older adults can take as many classes as they wish, in such subjects as the arts, history, the humanities, computers, and health.

I asked the Skolniks how replicable their NORC was. After all, most of us don't live in communities with as rich a tradition of cooperation as Greenbelt has. "If there's a sense of community and the political will, it's replicable," said Steve. "There's a very high level of services, but we pay for that through high taxes. There has to be a level of willingness on behalf of leaders to make the investment."

"A government structure to help provide services is more likely to succeed than if a developer did it," Lola said.

To them, the idea of living in Greenbelt is far more appealing than moving to a planned retirement community. "I like the idea of living in a *real* community," said Lola. "These senior living facilities have their place, but it's just for one strata."

"They're not appealing to me," said Steve, then laughs. "But maybe I'll get crotchety and won't want to be around kids."

"I love the idea of living in a place where there may be support services where I'd not have to move," Lola added.

☙❧

That Lola has that option is due to the foresight of the older generation nearly fifteen years ago. The spirit of working for the common good came through when the town was faced with the realization that many of its citizens were choosing to age in Greenbelt. In 1999, when the town's only nursing home closed, the city council decided it needed to determine how well Greenbelt's older residents were being served. The town had a HUD-supported affordable apartment building for seniors called Green Ridge House. They wondered if perhaps Greenbelt should look into having an assisted living center built as well. They formed a task force comprised of older people and three consultants to research the next step. The task force conducted surveys and held focus groups of older residents, family caregivers, and local businesses and agencies. After eighteen months of study, "The overwhelming response of citizens was, we want to stay in our homes, we want to age in place—you're going to have to take me out in a box," recalled Christal Batey, then one of the consultants, who is now Greenbelt's Community Resource Advocate.

In response to that sentiment, instead of a bricks-and-mortar building Greenbelt set up a NORC-SSP, a wide-ranging service program called Greenbelt Assistance in Living (GAIL) for people who are older or have disabilities. To develop GAIL, the city partnered with Greenbelt Housing, Inc., a cooperative of townhouse homeowners, such as the Skolniks, and applied for financial help from NORC Supportive Services, Nat Yalowitz's outfit up at Penn South. With a $136,579 grant, they hired the first community resource advocate in 2001. Christal came on board in 2003.

I met Christal in the municipal center, a two-story brick office building that straddles a parking lot between the New Deal Café and the community center. Her office, filled with notebooks, flyers, and pictures of her family, overlooks Crescent Drive, the main thoroughfare for old Greenbelt.

Reflecting on her early days in the job, Christal, a self-described "big believer in data," was anxious to have a needs assessment conducted. "If you listen to what people say, you get buy-in," she said. "People know what they need." Those needs were captured in a five-inch-thick binder handed to Christal by the consultant hired to conduct the assessment. The top five concerns of the older people in town were transportation; health care, particularly home-care; home safety and maintenance; information about available services; and finances, especially related to prescription drug costs. Armed with that knowledge, Christal designed a blueprint for moving forward. She must have done her job right: a decade later, GAIL serves nearly nine hundred people—up from eighty-five when she began her job a decade earlier. The cost, primarily for staff salaries, was $190,400 in the 2013 town budget.

"One thing that was paramount was that residents needed information," she said. "They wanted something better than opening up the yellow pages. We empower them through knowledge of what's out there and how to access it."

GAIL was formed around the same time as Beacon Hill Village. While both Villages and NORCs have the same goal of supporting people who want to stay rooted in their communities as they age, there are some key differences. "A Village is a private-pay version of what we have," said Christal. With city funds, GAIL supports every older person in the town, unlike most Villages, which support only their dues-paying members. (All-volunteer Villages are exceptions, e.g. Bannockburn's Neighbors Assisting Neighbors in Chapter 3.) "Because it's your tax dollars, everyone is eligible," she said. "I like the concept that everyone on the block can call for services, instead of Bob can call and Mary can't call because she's not a member."

The other advantage, she points out, is that the cost is picked up by the city and shared among all the taxpayers, rather than constantly having to raise funds, recruit members, and collect dues, as most Villages do.

GAIL, like Penn South Program for Seniors, provides care coordination or case management, which most Villages do not. (Capitol Hill Village is one of the exceptions.) GAIL also offers mobile counseling, free community nursing, home visits for everything from bathing to blood sugar monitoring, and patient advocacy during physician appointments.

Christal thought that for many Greenbelt residents, paying for such services would be prohibitive, or at least a deterrent. Calling herself the "Queen of Free," she said, "I don't want my people to pay for things that can be provided for free." She reached out to Bowie State University and Washington Adventist University nursing schools and set up a partnership whereby nursing students provide services for free, as part of their community nursing rotation. Medical students from Georgetown University School of Medicine also conduct visits in the community during their geriatrics rotation. Christal's hidden agenda is not only to get free services but also to expose the med students to older people, help them learn a good bedside manner, and maybe even entice them to specialize in geriatrics.

This program morphed into Health Assessment and Services (HAS), combining social work, public health, nursing, and therapeutic recreation—in short, many of the components of a nursing home—all provided by interns and overseen by clinical instructors. "The idea is that being *pro*active is better than *re*active," Christal said. "If we could put something in place that was preventative *in their home*, it might keep people from having to move."

GAIL also received grants to help people make their homes accessible, changing tubs to wheel-in showers, for example, or installing handrails or stair lifts, especially important since the original homes had no bathroom on the first floor. Residents who qualified could receive up to $5,000 to make home improvements that would allow them to remain independent. Because the grant was a federal Community Block Grant through HUD, the funds were restricted to those of modest means, unlike most GAIL programs, which are available to all.

GAIL has done a remarkable job of partnering with other agencies and schools to provide free services for older people as well as for Greenbelt residents generally. Recent programs include a community health fair, a community flu clinic, mental health screening day, memory screening day, door-to-door wellness assessments at Green Ridge House, and a Medicare lecture series, as well as free produce distribution: the Capital Area Food Bank donates the fruits and vegetables, and Greenbelt volunteers help with distributing it to any resident who shows up at a local elementary school or at Green Ridge House. The City also partnered with Prince George's County Department of Social Services to set up a satellite office in the municipal center so that residents would not have to travel to larger county buildings and wait in long lines. "Our building is one-stop shopping," Christal said. "We had to build those partnerships. We realize there's a limit to what volunteers can do. You can't ask volunteers to help bathe someone. Our partnership enable us to make services available."

"We can do as much or as little as you need," she said. "The thing that's important is that you become familiar with us when you don't need help so that when you do need us, you know who to call."

I asked her if older people in Greenbelt had a sense of ownership of GAIL, the way members of Villages do. How does she avoid having people feel like social service recipients, rather than empowered? "We constantly do satisfaction surveys and focus groups. Once a year there's a senior forum, organized by residents." City staff who interact with older people come and listen to people's gripes and kudos. "We're constantly seeking feedback," she said. "Residents feel that we hear them—that's what's important. The services are tailored to the client, and residents see themselves as individuals."

For a NORC (or a Village or any other such model) to truly be a different animal altogether than a social service agency, older people themselves must be in leadership and control. Greenbelt did that by putting older people in charge of the task force that led to GAIL's formation. Tom White, in his late seventies, headed up the task force back in 1999. He dubs Christal "Mrs. Aging-in-Place." He and his wife, Helen, have lived in Greenbelt more than fifty years. "Helen and I are very fortunate," he said. "Both of us are able-bodied. I guess we did have one eye on the future though." Like Lola Skolnik, the

Whites know that if they ever do have health problems, enough services are in place that they might be able to remain in the community they love.

Contributing to the community through meaningful volunteer work is another obvious way to break down the stereotype of older people being passive recipients of services. As one study notes, "a dynamic process should focus less on the social structure of organizations that serve elders and more on informal groups (neighbors helping neighbors) who support each other. *The advantage of this paradigm shift is to see elders as valuable assets rather than problems.* Because of their experiences, elders bring positive influences to younger generations in their communities; thus, they should play a greater role in shaping their environment and social networks" (emphasis added).[14]

In Greenbelt such a process is carried out by another important program initiated by residents called GIVES, for Greenbelt Intergenerational Volunteer Exchange Services. GIVES is a membership organization that nurtures a neighbors-helping-neighbors philosophy, primarily aimed at helping older people remain in Greenbelt. Some 220 members provide services to each other, with eight hundred services volunteered annually. Seventy percent of the members are older people.

The most frequent requests are for transportation (within a ten-mile radius). In addition, members ask for help with yard work, light housework, computer problems, and dog walking. Pairs of members are linked as calling buddies, to check on each other once a day.

"The majority of our members either receive services or give services, but you can work it both ways," explained Jean Cook, seventy-two, GIVES president. "I've been doing this for twelve or thirteen years, and I'm at the point in my life where I don't need it, so I give. But I needed help with my computer, so I called and someone came for a couple hours, and she received credit for those two hours."

Although GIVES tracks the hours, like a job bank, there is no quid pro quo. Jean estimates she's donated two thousand hours over the years, and the two hours of computer help was all she'd received.

Because the program is all volunteer, GIVES needs only in-kind help from the city. They have a nook off the senior lounge in the community center, and the city pays for a separate telephone line. GIVES accepts donations to pay for postage and toner for the computer printer. The biggest help from the city, though, is that GIVES volunteers are covered under the city of Greenbelt's insurance plan.

"Greenbelt by its nature has always been the kind of place where people volunteer to help one another," Jean said. "It's the way it's operated for seventy-five years. [My husband and I] were planning to stay a year or two and we've lived here forty-one years. We moved into our home and eight months after, our house was gutted by fire. Luckily we just had two children, and we each got out one of our little boys. Greenbelt took care of us. We received so much of an outpouring of kindness, and I said I guess we're staying here."

Today, she and her husband have no plans to ever leave. "We're here to stay because we love it," she said. "Greenbelt was a wonderful place to raise children, and it's a wonderful place to grow old."

✆

One challenge Christal is determined to tackle is adapting GAIL to meet the needs of the next generation of elders, the baby boomers. To that end, in 2010, she and her counterpart in the recreation department conducted a survey of the town's boomers. "How do they access services; how do they use technology?" Christal wondered. Baby boomers are a different breed than the Depression-era elders she has been serving. "[Boomers] don't want to be called 'seniors' or 'silver' this or that," she said. "They just want to be alive, not categorized."

The survey was initially prompted by the recreation department staffer wanting to know how to improve the lunch program to attract younger residents. The point of the lunch program is less about nutrition than about people having a chance to socialize. While many of the residents in their late seventies and eighties have been drawn by the virtually free (a donation is asked) lunch, the idea of a "congregant" meal of roast beef, mashed potatoes, and peas at the community center was not exactly a draw to people in their sixties.

"They're telling us, 'We don't want to go to a nutrition site. We'll go to a WIFI café,'" Christal said. "It's not your Mom's senior center that they want to go to. This is a generation that goes to Starbuck's and orders whatever they want—low sodium, gluten-free, whatever." But as the boomer generation grows old, she said, many of us caught with evaporating nest eggs and no pensions may change. That free lunch may look more appetizing. "You never know," she said. "People's perspective changes."

An example of what the coming generation of elders wants may be Susan Harris, a sixty-something self-employed gardening blogger, who recently moved to Greenbelt from my hometown of Takoma Park. During the twenty-six years she'd lived there, she had converted a large portion of her yard into garden beds. But she began to notice that when she looked out on her pride and joy, she began to feel burdened rather than blessed. She didn't feel close to many of her neighbors, who were mostly young families with children. The decision to sell her home was surprisingly easy, she said, helped by the fact that the buyers loved the garden.

She briefly considered moving to a traditional retirement community, but it didn't feel like the right fit. "I couldn't see myself in a golfing community of Republicans," as she imagined it. She had several criteria in her search for a place to move: low crime, walkable, comfortable, and affordable.

Although Greenbelt cooperative homes (Greenbelt also has houses that are not part of the cooperative) sell at market rate, they have traditionally cost less than many of the other Washington close-in suburbs. Most co-op homes are small, with a single bathroom on the second floor. They are also attached, with small yards and no garages.

As much as affordability, Susan wanted a place where being actively involved was the norm. "People move here who want to be part of the community," she said. "People expect that you'll volunteer on something. We have the oldest volunteer-published community newspaper in the country."

Just five months after moving there, she was already writing for the paper, and she'd offered to help put the news up on the web. She had hopes of starting a blog, with stories, photos, and videos of local goings on.

Now she has much less home and yard maintenance and lives on a quiet court. Her next-door neighbor is a single woman her age, and Susan hopes to make new friends soon, in addition to a few she had before moving there. She had already staked out a plot in the community garden and was exploring the free fitness classes offered to people over sixty.

Susan's decision to move not to a retirement community but to an age-friendly town like Greenbelt epitomizes what many of us will want.

I asked Jean Cook if she knew anyone in Greenbelt who had made the choice to move to a retirement community. She seemed horrified at the thought. Not a soul. "We joke about it," she said. "I always say I'm staying in Greenbelt until I go to Johns Hopkins—I've donated my body to science."

Tom White feels the same way. Reflecting on a large developer-built retirement community he visited in Florida, he said, "Practically everybody has a golf cart. There was a huge competition for how snazzy can your golf cart be. There's golf, there's swimming pools. Practically every night there's an outside social thing, a happy hour, music group—these people are doing very well there. But to me it was kind of sterile—it's a beautiful place and has a lot of activities, but it was like make-believe. I'd pick Greenbelt over that any day."

CHAPTER 7

Community Without Walls
Weaving a Web of Friendship

In 1992, Vicky Bergman, then forty-eight, began to contemplate her future. She and her husband, Dick, had been helping out his parents, who were in their eighties and having a difficult time with illness and frailty. She and Dick began to wonder what their own old age would be like.

After Dick's father died, his mother grew increasingly depressed and lonely. "Mom fell apart after being a caregiver to Dad," reflected Dick. His mother immediately moved in with Dick and Vicky, and six months later they found what they hoped would be a good situation for her, in a continuing care retirement community. But "she was never happy," Dick said.

Vicky and Dick took his parents' experience to heart and thought about how they could make their own old age different. They knew they wanted to remain in their home in Princeton, New Jersey. They also were smart enough to realize that without forethought, they were at risk of ending up alone and isolated.

The couple, more intentional than most, attended the Omega Institute Conference on Conscious Aging in New York, along with another couple from Princeton. Although they found the conference to be worthwhile, "We felt something was missing," said Vicky.

During this time, as she wrote later, they wrestled with their concerns—the fear of aging alone, the need for widening their friendship network when their longtime friends moved away or died, and the need for improving housing options and community infrastructure to meet the needs of older people in Princeton.[1]

To address these issues, the two couples, along with two other friends, decided to engage people they knew in a conversation about growing older. They sent out what became known as "the Falling Leaves letter" to their networks. The letter, an invitation to come to the Bergmans for coffee and conversation, began:

> With the start of the fall season many people think of a year coming to an end, and as we get older, there is frequently a bit of unease along with the falling leaves.

What lies ahead? Will I be well enough to live as I do now and, if so, for how long? Is my family nearby? Do I have friends younger than I am? Will I be able to stay in my own home?

Instead of just brushing these questions aside, a few of us got together to talk about a nurturing community of support—support that would allow us to stay in our own homes as long as we possibly could. Our experience with parents, other relatives, and friends, has brought the need to prepare for these pending problems into sharp focus.

We think you might be one of the people or couples who would be interested in pursuing the possibility of creating a nurturing "community without walls." The goal is to get rid of the fear and worry and to answer the quest of "who will be there for me?"[2]

They had hoped for a turnout of thirty or so, but twice that number crammed into the Bergman home, with participants ranging in age from forty-eight to ninety-two. "We were all talking about what we wanted and trying to pin down what was missing and suddenly I realized, this is it. The medium is the message," recalls Vicky, then the youngest of the group. In other words, the very act of talking and sharing and building relationships with each other was the missing piece.

From that emerged the Community Without Walls, Inc., a flourishing nonprofit that today has 450 people aged fifty and older from the Princeton area, organized into six chapters called Houses.

Houses meet monthly or quarterly, depending on the House. In addition, each House has small groups of members who share an interest, such as a walking club or book group. "Some are organized to build community," Vicky explained.

For example, people break into dyads, interview each other, and introduce each other to the whole group. Or you bring in a photo of a grandparent, and in a small group, each person talks about the photo. That helps us build connections and learn about our past. Most of us don't have friends from childhood around. Some people have those kinds of connections in the community, but many of us do not. How do you make those kinds of deep connections? The way is by doing things together.

I went to Princeton to attend a monthly gathering of the original group, known as House 1, and to meet the Bergmans and other members. Princeton has the feel of a charming historic village. If there's a wrong side of the tracks, I never saw it. On a late autumn day, the main street, near the campus of Princeton University, was filled with people lining up at restaurants and shopping.

The Bergmans live in an attractive neighborhood of solid homes just minutes from downtown. Evidence of the destructive force of Hurricane Sandy was everywhere, although the storm had passed through weeks earlier. Piles of brush and limbs were stacked along curbs.

Dick, a short man with white hair and a trim moustache, met me at the door and led me into their spacious bright kitchen. Vicky soon joined us. In her late sixties, she was youthful and stylish, with round-framed glasses, a bright-orange Derby hat, tapestry jacket, and chunky jewelry. The couple had done a stint in Washington, working in the Carter administration, and had a comfortable and full retirement, sharing CWW leadership and gourmet cooking, among many other activities.

We had a Sunday brunch of dim sum at a Chinese restaurant in the Princeton Shopping Center. This looked to be an ordinary strip mall, but, like much of Princeton, the shopping center is exceptional—the oldest one in New Jersey, I was told. Everything about Princeton seemed exceptional: it is exceptionally historic, settled by Quakers in 1636. It is exceptionally prosperous, with median income of $106,000, nearly twice that of New Jersey as a whole, and exceptionally educated, with faculty and many alumni from the famed Ivy League school.

"Princeton is the kind of place where everyone has two-and-a-half degrees and we think we know better than everybody else," quipped Dick. (In truth, they are an erudite bunch, and I found myself consulting the dictionary more than once after even brief conversations with CWW members.)

As we chatted over pig's ears, dumplings, and scallion pancakes, Vicky, Dick, and then–CWW president Ruth Randall filled me in on the organization's growth and its challenges.

CWW's initial and primary focus is to nurture relationships, they explain. Clearly, that must have struck a chord with the older crowd in Princeton, given the organization's steady growth.

Within five years one hundred people had joined, and the leaders had capped membership based on research that showed that larger groups have a harder time creating a strong sense of community among their members. As the waiting list grew, the idea of forming new chapters or Houses took hold.

In 1995 CWW incorporated as a 501(c)(3) nonprofit, both to protect members who may be hosting events at their homes from litigation if someone fell on their sidewalk, say, and to keep control over who uses the CWW name. New Houses are given charters to make sure the organization stays true to its original mission, although Houses create their own rules and plan their own events. House 3, for example, allows people to join after simply coming to a monthly meeting twice, while House 1 requires new members to be sponsored by current members.

The experience of Eunice, a member of House 2, is a good example of what CWW founders hoped to accomplish. In an email, she wrote:

> "Creating Community" is exactly what CWW, House 2 has been for me. When my husband passed away in 2002 a few years after joining the group, I found myself "wrapped around" with friendship and support. My three children all live out of state and out of concern for me were about to take charge of my life. For them, seeing the community-wide network of friends was reassuring. Everyone relaxed when seeing first hand that I wasn't stranded and alone. House 2 folks moved in with food and friendly attention. They helped coordinate a gathering at my house with my husband's university colleagues.

CWW had just celebrated its twentieth anniversary with a very successful conference when I visited. The conference attracted 255 participants, one-third of them non-members. Each House led a panel on a topic of its choice, which included building a successful aide/patient relationship, preparing for the inevitable (estate planning, grief, elder care), lifelong learning ("for the many opsimaths"—which, I learned, refers to those who like to learn late in life), poetry and aging, relationships across generations, aging and spirituality, and volunteerism.

During the conference Vicky heard many opinions—sometimes contradictory—on whether the organization was on the right track.

"Some people want more community-building stuff, not just social," she said. "They want it not so superficial."

"Others want more lectures," noted Ruth.

Dick opines that some (including him, I had the impression) dismiss "community building" as the "touchy-feely" stuff. But, he admitted, House 1, which began with more community-building than some other Houses, has been a great success. "Is it because it was started by people who were already friends?" he wondered. "Or is it because they did the touchy-feely stuff early on?"

I asked them how CWW differs from the Village model. "CWW is a bottom-up organization and members are expected to do what friends do," said Dick. "The Village is top down and provides services." While I doubt that Villages would describe themselves as "top down," I take his point, that Villages are a gateway of sorts to assistance, rather than essentially a network of friends.

Another significant difference is financial. Villages, as discussed in Chapter 3, typically charge dues that can sometimes amount to hundreds of dollars annually per person, primarily to cover an executive director and office space. In contrast, CWW's annual dues are $30, to cover the cost of the website, room rentals for large gatherings, and other incidentals. All help is volunteer and informal.

CWW leaders are adamant that what the organization provides is friendship, ensuring that no members grow old isolated and alone. They are also clear about what CWW is not: a service provider. They don't want to regard their members as "clients" but as friends. At the same time, as many of the members have gotten into their eighties and nineties, the issue of supportive services inevitably arose.

"Ten years ago we had a conference asking what was needed if we were to stay in our homes, and out of that conference came the idea for a nonprofit organization which could supply physical help—health care managers, and home health care aides, and the like," recalled Hilly, who has been a member for eighteen years.

To address such concerns Ruth Randall and other CWW leaders initiated a spin-off called Secure@Home. Just as CWW describes itself as a community of friends, Ruth compares Secure@Home to having "a useful daughter in town."

I later called Judy Millner, a geriatric care manager, registered nurse, and director of Secure@Home. As she recalled, "CWW put together a group that was considering as they age in place what their needs might be. They determined that neighbor supporting neighbor would only go so far when they were at a point where they needed more professional services. You can't have someone with cognitive impairment driving someone with a fractured hip. They put together a group that researched various agencies in the area and what they could provide." Jewish Family & Children's Services, with a seventy-five-year history working with older adults, was selected to run the new entity.

For a $400 annual fee ($450 per couple), Secure@Home staff conduct a comprehensive needs assessment and offer a number of services, including care management, twenty-four-hour on-call emergency telephone support, wellness classes, monthly phone check-ins, and vetting of vendors and providers.

For a nominal additional fee, Millner manages a client's medications, visiting twice a week to fill a pill dispenser. "Once we do the medication management and the compliance improves, we're actually able to make med adjustments so we might be able to take some of the meds away, because the blood pressure lowers or the situation is under control," she said. While she is there, she also checks the client's vital signs and is able to troubleshoot any problems early on.

As the program has evolved, an older and frailer population is joining; the average age of its 230 members is eighty-one, with many people in their nineties. Nevertheless only 7 percent of Secure@Home clients have had to move from their homes over the past six years. The organization has also made great strides in reducing readmissions to hospitals, a growing and costly concern for Medicare. Millner has come to believe that with the right resources—including financial, it's important to note—most people can remain in their own homes until the end.

Fran, seventy-nine, a founding member of House 3, describes Secure@Home as "an insurance policy unlike any other that I have—as long as I live, they're going to help me. I think Secure@Home is doing a beautiful job." She appreciates the monthly calls to make sure she's doing okay, and she's taken advantage of the organization's Chore Corps, a team of volunteers who help with everyday tasks. "I bought a new desktop computer, and a guy must have spent two hours installing it," she said. "Then he took and gave away the old one. They are very caring people." Secure@Home thus combines the practical help of a Village with more professional services offered through many NORCs.

Another change that has occurred since CWW's founding is that there are more options for retirement communities and assisted living than there were in 1992. In fact, despite its main emphasis on aging in place, CWW has pushed for more living options for older people and initiated the Coalition for Senior Housing in Princeton.

A small number of CWW members have chosen to leave their own homes. In a 2011 survey of House 2, for example, of fifty-five who responded, six had moved. Two of these members (one couple) downsized to a smaller home that was in walking distance of the center of town, and four others moved to a Princeton retirement community. People who moved said they did so because of deteriorating health, the burden of home upkeep, growing tired of cooking, or wanting to be near more peers.

When people move out of their homes, the experience is mixed as to whether they remain involved in CWW. "What happens is, we become connected to the members of our House," said Vicky. "If they move to assisted living and aren't driving, someone will pick them up and bring them to the meetings. If they're in the dining group, someone will say, 'Martha's got to be picked up.' And that's the way it works." Others told me that when people move to a retirement community or assisted living they become involved in their new communities and drift away from CWW.

❧

Later that afternoon, I accompanied the Bergmans to House 1's monthly gathering, held in a renovated barn that was once part of the Robert Wood Johnson estate and is now parkland. A large upstairs room was set up with rows of chairs, a lectern, and tables for members to set out goodies to share.

"The main thing about CWW is eating," joked long-time member Judith Pinch. Judith, like many CWW members, is intellectually active and a lifelong learner. She is a founder of the Evergreen Forum, which offers peer-led courses to adults. A recent semester of nineteen courses included everything from "Opera Potpourri" to "Global Political Economy," "5000 Years of Chinese History & Culture," and "Encountering Kafka." "CWW is important for us, but the intellectual stimulation from Evergreen is even more important," she said.

Two friends, Helen and Pei, joined CWW when House 1 had some openings. Both women lived alone and appreciated being part of a supportive community. Without CWW, said Helen, "If you're not well, who would you call? Who would you ask? Everybody will pitch in here."

Pei offered a common refrain: "We're all so proud and don't want anybody to do anything for us."

"With this group, we can ask," Helen said. "One of the biggest problems of older people is the sense of isolation."

Pei added that the lectures and support have made her feel more comfortable with the whole notion of aging in place. She also joined Secure@Home and was pleased that during Hurricane Sandy someone called to check on her safety.

Both women felt that CWW also advocated for their interests, raising the need for senior housing and transportation options in Princeton, for example.

Helen, a published poet who used to teach writing to women employees at Princeton University, has led groups on poetry and on memoir writing for CWW. The latter opened her eyes to the diversity of backgrounds of other members. A Boston native, Helen enjoys the stories from new friends who grew up in such exotic places as Montana and the Bahamas. Sharing their memoirs brought their small group closer.

Mort, the vice-president of House 1, is one of many who told me that

CWW "opens up pathways to meeting people you'd otherwise not meet." People who have lived in Princeton half-a-century are suddenly exposed to a much wider circle than they even knew existed in their town.

I heard this from several members. Eunice wrote: "Action bubbles up from the diversity. Activity groups form within the House and that cements the social connections. House 2 has a very active thespian group that has a great time with play reading. . . . I started a walking group. . . . As a large group, House 2 meets about five times per year. Our meetings are primarily social and sometimes we have speakers of interest. We also have potluck sign-up lunches and dinners. Fun seems to be our primary goal. We try to keep organizational tasks to a minimum. CWW has truly enriched my life."

Others mentioned they saw homogeneity more than diversity. The organization is mostly white (even more so than Princeton as a whole), highly-educated, and prosperous. This is no surprise, perhaps, as the main way of growing is word of mouth with friends inviting friends to join.

Merle, program coordinator for House 4, started a Women In Transition (WIT) group that was so popular it mushroomed into three groups. Among the many topics they've discussed are your mother's relationship with money, what part did music play in your life, hair ("we got some really amazing responses"), and remembering and forgetting. "It's not set out to be a support group, but just hearing other people's stories that mirror your own is very supportive," she said.

One creative offshoot of CWW is a drama group called On Stage, which draws participants from across Houses. Describing itself as documentary theater, the group takes people's stories related to a theme, such as family or the experience of learning something new, reworks them and gives them shape, and then presents them as a dramatic performance. The group also does intergenerational performances, and they are receiving training in dramatic techniques.

At the House meeting, On Stage actor Ruth pulled me aside to tell me about the project and to ask me to send them good stories that I come across. "We're always looking for material," she said. On Stage has been an amazing experience for her, a chance to explore a creative part of herself that she never knew existed. "To do improv is wild," she said. "It keeps stretching me. It's such a wonderful thing."

One small group that delves deeply into personal concerns is House 2's "Death and Dying" group, affectionately known as D&D. D&D organizer Claire joined CWW nearly twenty years ago, in her late fifties. One of House 2's first efforts was to encourage members to complete advance directives (living wills). Claire noticed that most of the women had no hesitation filling out the forms, but many of the men were less willing. "I thought, these people need to talk about death," she recalled. "So I said 'anybody who wants to talk about death and dying can come to our house. We'll have a brown bag lunch and we'll talk about it.'" She felt initially, "Everybody looked at me as if I'd crawled out from under a brick." But she ended up with thirty people crowded around their dining room table. "It was astounding," she said. "People were willing to talk about this but they wanted a smaller venue."

The group split in half, to encourage conversation. "It's not everybody's cup of tea by any manner of means," she said. "I thought we'll [meet] five or six times. Then I mentally brushed my hands" (having finished the job). And yet, two decades later, they're still meeting, having settled into a close-knit group of a dozen or so. They discuss everything from funeral directors and "the obscenity of caskets—the ones made of mahogany and gold inlay," to advance directives, the one child who "refuses to pull the plug," and how to transition to living alone after the death of your spouse.

"It is a place to come with one's most intimate fears, concerns, angers," she said. "We've had people more than once say, 'I'm so mad at him or her for dying.'"

At the same time, she said, "It is not at all grim—we laugh quite a lot. We are a mixed bag as far as religious belief or nonbelief. Interestingly we don't talk about life after death. We talk about philosophical and social problems. And we talk about trying to have a reasonable old age."

Perhaps most importantly, the group offers strong emotional support to those suffering loss, support that goes beyond what Claire calls "the line of chicken soup" showing up at your door. They stay attentive for months, rather than days. "We provide simple comfort," she said.

One of our members right now, her husband is terminally ill and deeply damaged. She comes when she can, and we say as much as we can. While he was still able to get around, various people would have them to dinner. It's interesting when people are seriously ill or in a wheelchair or beginning to have that very, very thin look—there are many, many people who find that terrifying, and we do not. I don't say that in a smug way. After a while we look beyond the impedimenta—so you're on oxygen, so you have a catheter, so what? If you looked at us, none of us look like the grim reaper is sitting in the living room!

The one thing this circle of people feels now is absolute freedom to talk about virtually anything, about their most intimate feelings about what it's like to lose somebody or face one's own demise. We give enough space and time, and we don't interrupt each other. It's amazing how comforting a quiet silence can be.

ᘒᘓ

Even as there are stirring testimonials like this one, there are of course challenges. "It's a paradigm shift," said Vicky. "We have to learn how to want support. People have to go in their brains and say, 'I have to reach out.'"

"Far more people are willing to provide help than ask for it," agreed Dick.

Ruth had been president of CWW for five years and had a long history of leadership, including being past president of the local teacher's union, yet she found it difficult to recruit committed volunteers for CWW. "Our trouble is getting leadership," she said. "People don't realize that to develop relationships, one way is to serve."

Dick said it's a classic example of the Pareto Principle, which states that with anything in life there's a 20-80 distribution. (I had to look that one up too—the principle stems from Vilfredo Pareto's observation in 1906 that 20 percent of Italians owned 80 percent of the nation's wealth and has since been applied to all sorts of phenomena.) Dick's point was that 20 percent of CWW members do 80 percent of the work, and that this is likely true for most organizations.

Another obstacle is that CWW chose to organize itself by chronology of membership: the longest-participating members are in House 1, and the newest members in House 6. As a result, people who live in the same neighborhood may well be in different Houses. Thus, carpooling or offering rides to those who can no longer drive is often unworkable. People may not know members who are in other Houses, even if they live nearby. "When [Hurricane] Sandy hit, we helped our neighbors, not CWW," said John, a retired minister and member of House 1. To bridge this gap, Ruth was working on a neighborhood cross-referenced list, to let members know if they live near someone else in CWW.

Within the organization there also seems to be a tension between those who want more organized support in times of need versus those who would prefer that such support evolve organically among those individuals who develop a close bond. Houses have organized buddy systems whereby members help someone through a crisis by organizing meals, transportation, or visits. But not everyone feels the need to use the system, said Merle, program director of House 4. For example, she would likely call on her daughters who live nearby for support. Others say they would turn to family or long-time friends, rather than CWW.

John is cochair of the contact coordinators group in House 1. He's made a folder for each member that includes forms that give their contact coordinator permission to advocate on their behalf at the hospital. He said there was not agreement about the role of the care coordinators. Some see them as "first responders," who help during an emergency run to the hospital, at which point professionals and family members would take over. "But there was a time when we could visit and help people over an extended period," he said. Some feared, though, that raising such an expectation among members would be unrealistic and unsustainable. "The idea is if we're close enough that will happen anyway," he said.

He and others suggest other valuable things CWW could do. "Seniors tend to think the ideal is to mimic twenty-five-year-olds," he said. "We ought to promote what seniors are good at, like other cultures do. We should promote our wisdom."

Common problems, such as planning to transition from a house that is far too big for an older single person, or paring down and organizing belongings, often go unaddressed, say others.

"I think CWW could do a great deal more of activism—political and otherwise—as a large consumer organization, in transportation, in medical matters such as improving the provision of home care aides," said Hilly of House 2. "But there has been strong resistance to that sort of talk."

Although some of the members I meet find that CWW fills an important niche in their lives, others seem to be natural "joiners" and not in need of yet another social group. Burt and Roberta, a handsome and active couple, hardly seem to need community. She's a social worker and he is an extremely busy volunteer—raising funds for prostate cancer; tutoring in English as a second language; working in Parks and Recreation—and both are active in their synagogue. They moved from their own home to an "adult" community. "We wanted to be near Princeton," Roberta said. "We love taking courses and the arts. We made some friends and joined a bridge group." When Sheilah, the president of House 1, invited her to join, Roberta asked why? In other words, what would be the point, given her full life?

"Sheilah said you can never have too many friends," Roberta recalled.

She and Burt plunged in, joining the movie group and the eating-out group, and Roberta even serves on the CWW steering committee. Yet despite this level of commitment, she does not think of CWW as her primary support system. "If I had a crisis would they be the people I call?" she demurred. "I don't have the history."

I realize the organization means different things to different people, and that may be a good thing. Many CWW members like Burt and Roberta are actively involved in other organizations and seem to already have strong social networks. For them, CWW programs—lectures, films, book clubs and so on—are appealing and enriching. Others, especially those who are single, value the friendship and support more. For her part, Ruth Randall sees CWW members as "in between friends and acquaintances. You can call on people for support."

Roberta mused that CWW may need to evaluate its reason for being. "To me it's fascinating," she said. "Will it last?"

❧

That question has some potency: I heard repeatedly from members that CWW was having a hard time attracting baby boomers. "And that's important," said Merle, "because if we don't get younger people we're going to die and it's a shame because it's such a great organization." The bulk of the members are in the seventy to eighty-five range.

"It's a problem having an older cohort," said Ruth. "People can't volunteer as much or accept leadership."

Betsy is one of the small number of people in their sixties who have joined in recent years. "I was a bit taken aback by being so much younger," she said of her introduction to CWW. Yet she and her husband are glad they joined. "I found a community of people who had done very interesting things with their lives in a world I hadn't traveled in. I found them engaging and kind and many of them of my background, which is Jewish. So I kept going. My husband seemed to enjoy them—we were the only ones that were younger, so he had some reservations at first. It's been three years now."

She wonders whether CWW will succeed in attracting others her age. "We don't do a good job recruiting younger members," she said. "We don't know how to. When [younger] people do come they look around and move on. Also the people who are there have a level of comfort with people they know. When I called about a movie group, I was told it was closed." The group goes to dinner afterward, the table was full, and they didn't want to expand to a second table. "It's an odd thing," she said. "They want younger people, but they also are hesitant about letting you in."

But perhaps most significant is another of her observations: twenty years is quite a difference in age. Although she appreciates and enjoys being with older people, she wonders if her peers would. She maintains an active fitness regime, for example, one that might be too strenuous for many of her CWW friends. "Everyone moves pretty slowly; and there are—as you would expect in a very senior age group—a number of canes, walkers, and hearing aids. I may be evaluated for one soon!" she said.

Her perspective made me wonder if the artificial age our society has set for "old" is simply too long a time period, now that people are living so long. Does it make sense for people twenty or thirty years apart in age to be viewed as the same cohort? This came about in large part because of external structures and benefits programs—from Social Security and Medicare to AARP membership and senior discounts on everything from airfare and movies to "early-bird specials" at the local diner—which lump sixty-five-year-olds or even younger in the same category as a ninety-year-old, based on what was once the traditional retirement age. In fact, those are two separate generations—and might easily encompass parents and children, not just peers.

This issue is not unique to CWW. Many other communities with older people as their constituency, from traditional retirement communities to elder cohousing and the Penn South Program for Seniors struggle to attract those in their sixties or even seventies. If a group becomes comprised almost entirely of the "oldest-old," the younger will be unlikely to join, thus threatening the organization's future as well as losing a source of healthier, fitter volunteers to help the older members.

Surprisingly, given its longevity and growth, CWW has not been replicated, as far as its founders know. They've responded to many inquiries from people in other towns and have done a lot of public speaking. But as far as they know, nothing has stuck. Princeton elders may be an unusually sophisticated, highly educated bunch, but the Community Without Walls model certainly seems adaptable to all sorts of demographics: it's inexpensive, easy to organize, and might be especially good for folks who don't have a "ready-made" community through a congregation or neighborhood. Yet few outside Princeton know of its existence—which seems a shame. Members I spoke to said they value its presence in their lives.

"There is a gallantry about CWW, and I don't mean that in a condescending way at all," said Claire. "If you come to a gathering or a party, certainly the brown bag lunch, everybody wears their best, looks their best, is their best. Everyone shows a gallantry about sailing out without complaint, of putting one's best foot forward in a community that I think is a very touching and strong thing. That is one thing that CWW is very good at."

CHAPTER 8

Generations of Hope
Living Well by Doing Good

It's not everyone who decides to move in retirement from San Diego to Rantoul, Illinois, to live in a community built on an abandoned military base. But such was the appeal of Hope Meadows that Clarissa did not hesitate to relocate from sunny Southern California to the small town Midwest, where winter's average low is in the teens.

"This was so attractive to me and I don't plan to ever leave," Clarissa said of her new life. "This is my last home."

What drew her to Rantoul was a community that surely ranks as one of the most inspiring places to settle. At Hope Meadows, she found a home for three key constituencies who often are marginalized: foster children who have been neglected or abused, their adoptive parents who lack support as they struggle to create a family, and elders who are looking for a sense of meaning and purpose.

"What we're working towards is a whole new way of life to support vulnerable people," said Brenda Eheart who founded Hope Meadows in 1994. "Another way of putting it is to really have ordinary people help solve these intractable social problems—that's what it's about."

Brenda founded Hope Meadows after growing increasingly frustrated with the failure of the foster care system to transform children's lives. Too often children are shuffled from family to family, while overwhelmed adoptive parents are often ill-equipped to handle the children's emotional and psychological problems. Brenda's solution was radical: to create normalcy for these troubled kids. From the ground-up she conceived of a nurturing community that was as normal as Mayberry, where kids felt safe and looked after by their parents and other caring adults.

To afford to create such a community, Brenda Eheart found property at the closed Chanute Air Force Base, a vast ghost town in need of new purpose. She initially envisioned houses for a small number of adopting families. But with so much housing available from the base closing, she ended up taking eighty homes and adding what became a core component: affordable housing for older people, thus bringing the steady hand and wisdom of elders to the mix. Today, Hope Meadows has forty-five older people and ten adoptive families with thirty-six kids, who are a mix of foster, adopted, and birth children.

In exchange for reduced rent—25 percent lower than market rate—older residents are expected to volunteer six hours each week in the community. Many volunteer more.

The adoptive parents receive a stipend from Hope Meadows, as payment for being "family managers," as well as free rent. To cover this, Hope Meadows receives funding through the state's foster care system. This makes it possible, with a modest lifestyle, for a single parent to remain at home to care for the children. In two-parent families, one usually has a job outside the home.

Driving through Rantoul, "You wouldn't know that you were in this special neighborhood," said Elaine Gehrmann, who took over as director of Hope Meadows in 2010. "Our housing looks much like the housing around us. We don't have a fence or gate or anything. That was the intention from the beginning—to not be removed from the rest of the community and not be designated as this place of old people and foster kids, but a regular neighborhood."

In age-restricted communities, she continued, "The seniors lose out. I think parents and kids do benefit greatly from the wisdom and experience and support of the older generation. It benefits all the generations. That's how human generations have been arranged for thousands of years, and we've gotten away from that. We've had to fill in with professional services and they're wonderful, but there's something about genuine, real intergenerational relationships that you're not paying for that professionals can't offer."

In the wonderful book *Hope Meadows: Real-Life Stories of Healing and Caring from an Inspiring Community*, former *Chicago Tribune* national correspondent Wes Smith told many heart-warming tales of these genuine relationships. One was of Esther, a widow who had lost her beloved husband of forty years, and who had since had serious and painful medical problems including two hip replacements, back surgery, and a heart by-pass operation. She found a new life at Hope Meadows. Smith quotes Esther:

> We have to just take [the children] as they come to us, and we run with them any way we can. You have to build trust. It's a wonderful thing to do. . . .
>
> I guess I love it here because there is something to get up for every morning. I like watching children develop. I like to feel like I'm helping with that. And I like that people honestly care about how you feel and about your well-being. It's meant a healthier life for me. No matter how much I hurt, I still get up and go because I know the children are waiting for me. If I get despondent or worried about something, there is always

some sort of pat on the arm. One little girl I was tutoring looked up at me the other day and said, "Why are you so grouchy?" She was right. I hadn't been feeling very well that day, but she made me laugh, so I wasn't grouchy anymore.[1]

That circle of caring and reciprocity is what has earned Generations of Hope, the nonprofit that operates Hope Meadows, international recognition and numerous awards, including being honored by the Congressional Coalition on Adoption Institute, the governor of Illinois, and the US Department of Health and Human Services, and chosen as a finalist by Harvard University for its Innovations in American Government Award. Brenda Eheart was elected an Ashoka Fellow for being one of the world's leading social entrepreneurs. The project also been widely covered in the press, from *NBC Nightly News* and *Oprah* to *USA Today*, *AARP The Magazine*, and the *New York Times*, where Clarissa first read about it in 2007.

"Hope is so organized," she said, and that made her transition easy. "They have a welcoming committee, and immediately people start coming over to help you and take you to lunch. I didn't have a car for a couple of weeks, and people took me grocery shopping. They have everything set up here."

Clarissa had a wealth of experience to bring with her. In the early 1970s she had lived in an intentional community of three hundred people. A registered nurse, she had founded a successful girl's empowerment project in San Diego that helped homeless girls and their chosen mentors—a teacher, mother, counselor, or other important woman in their lives—through a program of empowerment exercises and fun. "It was very satisfying, but something was missing," she said. "I was with them for a very short period of time—I wondered what happens with their lives later?" She longed for an opportunity to establish deeper relationships.

When she read about Hope Meadows, she was intrigued, but the time was not right for her to move. She was married to a retired professor who was very involved in the theater community and who had no desire to relocate to Rantoul. When he died suddenly of a heart attack, Clarissa was ready for a significant change in her life.

At Hope Meadows, she can afford a big house with plenty of room for an art studio—another one of her passions. Clarissa pays just $488 a month for a four-bedroom home that is more spacious than her $3,000 a month condo in San Diego.

For their required volunteer work, older people do whatever appeals to them, whether tossing a ball with kids, helping out in the office, or planting a garden. Clarissa helps with after-school activities for elementary school-aged children in the community. The kids work on art projects in her studio or do dance and movement with her.

"What I like best is I'm never lonely or bored," she said. "We have all kinds of scheduled weekly things: every Friday there's a potluck luncheon; we have a library, a computer center."

Another big plus, she said, is, the older people get special treatment—younger volunteers in the community shovel the snow, take the trash cans to the curb, and do minor home repairs.

David Netterfield and his wife Carol moved to Hope Meadows in 2008 out of a desire to do something good in the world. They had met through a Christian Singles online dating service, he in Wyoming and she in Chicago. They found they shared a desire to spend their next chapter on making a contribution. Carol had heard about Hope Meadows years ago on *Oprah*, and she suggested they consider it. They eventually got married and visited Hope Meadows several times before making the move.

David recalled one visit that clinched things. "One day about noon we were standing on the sidewalk in front of one of the adoptive family's homes and the thirteen-year-old son came home from school and came up and greeted his mom and us. He had never seen us before. His mom said these are the Netterfields and they're looking at possibly moving here. He said, 'Oh good. This apartment right here beside ours is vacant and has been for a while. Would you move in, so we could have some grandparents?'" David paused. "What can you do but get choked up?"

After moving there, the Netterfields ended up growing quite close to that family. When they learned that the mother needed transportation to get the boy to a special counselor, they volunteered to help out. They ferried the boy weekly, 150 miles round trip, eating at a restaurant after his counseling session before driving home. "We did this on our own, out of our own pocket, because we loved the little guy," he said. "By the time we'd done this for about a year, you can guess that we were pretty well attached to him."

This was the idea behind Hope Meadows—that relationships would grow naturally, out of affection rather than a sense of obligation or as a part of one's job. The kids, for their part, also help out in the community. David told of one family with seven children, three of them adopted from foster care. The mother herself had been in foster care as a teenager. "They've got two teenage girls that do a lot of babysitting and volunteer work around the Hope neighborhood," David said. "They just reach out and try and be helpful. They've grabbed on to every bit of goodness of this mother and dad and display it themselves with the Hope residents here. They walk dogs; they've helped seniors move in and unpack. At community gatherings that we have, they'll go down in the basement and babysit the younger children while the adults are upstairs."

Not that every story has a perfect ending. As David explained, the children arrive at Hope Meadows with fear and trepidation. Some have lived in over a dozen foster homes, and they assume this will be just another way station in their troubled lives. Many have been abused and most neglected. Some are so badly damaged they are unable to adjust to a normal family situation, even with all the counseling and support that Hope Meadows offers. "Sometimes there is a background that overwhelms both the adults and the youngster in the family and it doesn't work out," David said. "So occasionally the circumstances just kind of explode in everybody's face and break down and cease to be productive and it is deemed to be best for all parties concerned for the youngster to not be adopted and not stay here. It's heart breaking." Still, in the five years the Netterfields have been there, well over a hundred children have been successfully adopted and only a handful have had to return to the foster care system. Moreover, all the adopted children have gone on to graduate from high school or earn an equivalent certificate, compared to just 30 percent of children in the foster care system nationally.

"This is one of the finest social programs that I've ever been exposed to, with quite a real success rate," he said. "I'm proud to be a small part in what goes on here, and to do whatever I can to make things better for people's lives. It's not only reaching out and helping others—I see how it has had a positive impact in my own life as I try to live out my own Christianity."

I asked David how long he envisions remaining at Hope Meadows. "Until I die," he said without hesitation.

This lifelong commitment, not unusual at Hope Meadows, was unanticipated by the founders. As time has passed, residents who came in their sixties are now in their eighties and have no desire to move. Yet the old military base housing is not suited for frailty: the homes are two-story, with no bath on the first floor. To meet their needs and honor their wish to remain, Hope Meadows just invested in a new building, Hope House, for their oldest members who are unable to comfortably remain in their multi-story homes. Hope House, which opened in 2013, was built in the middle of the community to encourage interaction and connectedness. It has four single-floor apartments and one apartment for rehabilitation. "The idea is they don't have to go off and move somewhere," Elaine said. "They can continue to age in the center of community."

Because of Hope Meadows' success, in 2006 the Generations of Hope Development Corporation (GHDC) was created with funding from the W. K. Kellogg Foundation to spread the model throughout the nation. Led by

Brenda Eheart, GHDC has helped establish two more communities, Bridge Meadows in Portland, Oregon, and Treehouse in Easthampton, Massachusetts.

Bridge Meadows was built in an urban neighborhood in north Portland on a two-acre lot where a public school once stood. There are nine homes for adoptive families and twenty-seven apartments for low-income elders. The energetic founding director Derenda Schubert, a clinical psychologist, was inspired to develop Bridge Meadows after reading the *Hope Meadows* book. She had worked with children in the foster care system and felt that despite professionals' best efforts, the system was wanting. "I'd been watching these children languish in the foster care system and get mental health problems," she said.

> It's horrible. We did our best to help the children and I'm proud of the work we did, but I never thought we were doing enough. I wished they had a family that would love them forever, rather than all the counseling, the medication, all that we were trying to create, but then we'd go away. They still need someone to go home to at Christmas, to say, "Way to go" on that math paper, and someone to pick them up after sports practice. I felt that was missing.

At Bridge Meadows, which opened in April 2011, she has been astounded how quickly the children begin healing once they are adopted and settled into the community. The children become like cousins to one another, and having the common history of the foster care system creates a bond. "Watching them find their strengths and being celebrated for their accomplishments— or even, you got a new haircut and people notice," said Derenda. "They just start beaming. I have no doubt these kids are going to have wonderful lives, whether they become chefs or corporate executives or stay-at-home parents."

In fact, it is the older people who have had a tougher transition, according to Derenda. Unlike Hope Meadows, Bridge Meadows is designated as affordable housing, and to apply you must earn in the low $30,000s or less. Some of the older residents were hard-hit by the recession and the housing crisis, and they never imagined themselves needing affordable housing. Others arrive unsure of how they'll fit in with the younger families.

"The common denominator of our elders was anxiety," said Derenda.

> They were worried about their own situation. The nervousness started when they visited. They would think, "I see this community, I want it so badly." They were worried about their finances, and this could solve so many of their worries. It's a huge life transition—to move, exacerbated

when you're older and changing routines. They'll ask, "What is the rule?" We'll say, "Go be with the kids, go hang out with the moms." After they get their groove in—it takes about six months—they connect with the children, or they find their talent or where they're seen as the expert.

One decided to take on the newsletter and assigned children to be the reporters. Another is a natural-born storyteller and artist. She sits out on a bench in the middle of the community with paper and colored pencils and is soon surrounded by little kids wanting to draw.

The older residents pay about $500 a month in rent, and must complete a twenty-page application aimed at finding people who will be committed to the community. They are required to volunteer several hours a week and to suggest how they might contribute, as part of their lease. "The reason we put that in the lease is this idea of connection, that we were serious about that," she said. "We understood that isolation is one of the key elements of elders being ill and health issues going unnoticed. And children who have been in the foster care system and now in a family, they've been in situations of isolation too and that's how abuse is bred. This idea of connection we take quite seriously, based on scientific research that said how bad isolation is for you."

Derenda stresses that creating such a community requires an incredible amount of work and persistence, beginning with raising the money, designing the spaces, and overcoming "NIMBYism" (Not In My BackYard) among neighbors. She was proactive, inviting four people from the neighborhood to serve on the twelve-member design committee. Their input is reflected in many ways: Bridge Meadows has garages, paint colors that fit well with the surrounding neighborhood, a community building that does not look institutional, and a wide sidewalk that runs through the middle of the community, allowing outsiders to stroll through. The attitude went from "we don't need another social experiment here" to one of welcome. "They are pleased with us," she said. "They now hold their neighborhood meetings at Bridge Meadows. It was quite a journey."

The architectural and design team created spaces that would nurture interaction and community. In the center is a large vegetable garden and green space for the children to play. Benches are set strategically around the property to encourage the elders to sit and chat. A huge patio has furniture during the warm months, and there is a large community room and kitchen, a smaller community room for music and "toddler time," a library, computer room, and study room. A comfortable lobby near the mailboxes became a natural gathering spot.

Like Hope Meadows, the community is unusually diverse, with one third of elders coming from a community of color, over 70 percent of the children, and 40 percent of the adopting parents. The older members range in age from fifty-five to eighty-nine.

"Our eighty-nine -year-old moved to Bridge Meadows at the age of eighty-seven from Portland," said Derenda. "Her neighbors thought she was crazy. She'd always dreamed of such a community. Her daughter was connected to a donor, and she came to visit us. She said, 'I'm going to go get my mother' and left." The construction crew assumed she meant she'd return another day, but she returned that afternoon with her mother. The construction manager put hard hats on the women, and that was that.

"She's our wise sage," said Derenda. "Everyone is very respectful of her. We jokingly call her The Queen. She had a serious medical crisis, and we thought this would be the first person who we'd celebrate her life. But she's doing great. She's going to outlive me at this point."

ℰℱ

It's stories like these that motivate Brenda Eheart to keep on with the hard work of spreading a model that seems incredibly effective yet daunting to re-create. She is convinced that an intergenerational community, rather than an approach that is social-service or medically-based, can heal all sorts of people, not only foster children. Emerging efforts around the country based on the Generations of Hope model will center around different vulnerable populations: Wounded Warrior veterans, young mothers coming out of prison, or adults with developmental disabilities and their caregivers.

"The model is based on four key principles," Brenda explained.

- The community is composed of at least three generations
- The housing is contiguous
- The community is organized around a population of need
- The older adults volunteer in exchange for reduced housing costs

She expects that young retirees will make up one-half to two-thirds of a community's population.

Brenda, sixty-eight, is thinking more and more about the Hope Meadows model being used expressly to support frail elders. "I'm personally absolutely fascinated about growing old in community until the very end of life and still have meaning and purpose and really give back," she said.

Her latest vision is to have a community centered around perhaps ten elders with Alzheimer's disease or serious chronic conditions and their care-givers, who each have their own apartments. "Then you would have your boomers who are retiring who haven't become frail yet and who have energy and time—they would move there, and the idea would be to support the frail elders," she said. "And then you'd have ten households of young families and everybody would volunteer."

Brenda imagines such communities being built in small towns, next to public schools. The older people would go to the school to exercise or use computers. They'd also support school activities and sports and help tutor. Older people who had left the area for work might return, to find purpose and meaning in their retirement years, and younger families might stay rooted and able to obtain affordable housing.

With Bridge Meadows and Treehouse, Brenda has proven the model is replicable. Now she needs the funding and local leadership to spread it further.

 ෧౩

As inspiring as this model is, of course there are challenges. At Hope Mead-ows, as with any group of humans, people are not perfect. There is concern that some of the older residents move there primarily for the reduced rent, rather than to bond with children. There is not always as much closeness be-tween them and the parents as was intended. The community is trying differ-ent activities to try to bring people closer together.

Carol, seventy, who moved there two years earlier from Texas, said she was surprised and disappointed that many of the older people do not connect well with the kids. They hate the noise or the language the teens use. "I didn't ex-pect that," she said. "I expected that the only ones who would come here are those who really enjoyed children, and that was hard. They still do the volun-teering but not directly with the kids."

Carol, who worked with students with physical disabilities as a school physical therapist in El Paso before retiring, has always loved children and has a high tolerance for their shenanigans and noise. At Hope Meadows, two brothers, ages five and six, come to her house each week for four hours, and she enjoys taking kids on outings like to a pumpkin patch in the country. "I got quite close to one boy who is now thirteen and took him to gymnastics once a week," she said. "We're still friends and sometimes he'll come over on a Saturday and stay all day. I have family in Milwaukee and last year I took him to the state fair."

She also does a considerable amount of other volunteer work, taking the community's recycling into Champaign-Urbana, working in the Hope Meadows office, picking up donated bread from Panera for her neighbors, and helping with the community newsletter. "It makes for a busy life," she laughed.

Despite some disappointments, she has found a supportive, caring community within the elder population that she values. "It's not Nirvana," said Carol. "But I haven't had one moment that I was sorry I came here."

She shares a favorite anecdote. On a recent Saturday, the two little boys who regularly hang out at her house were sitting down to eat a meal with her. "I don't usually say grace, but one said, 'Can we hold hands and say grace?' I said of course, and he said 'Thank you God for the bestest day I ever had with a senior. And may it happen again.'"

CHAPTER 9

Affinity Groups
Settling with Your Tribe

In the 2012 film *Quartet*, directed by Dustin Hoffman, aging musicians live out their last years at Beecham House, a British retirement community set in a mansion on a lovely estate. Strains of violins, pianos, and operatic voices waft through the house and out across the expansive lawns as elders continue to practice their passion for music.

The longing to live in community with like-minded souls, the film suggests, runs deep. Even as tolerance and respect for diversity are on the rise in our multi-cultural world, many of us gravitate toward living with our "tribe," however we define that.

If you pull back the lens far enough to view the alternatives in this book, they generally reflect a desire to live around people with whom we have a bond, whether it's our neighbors in the Village, NORC, or cooperative; our friends or family with whom we share a house; or our cohousing comrades who seek to create an intentional community.

Although all retirement communities share the bond of same-age peers (if you call a span of thirty years or more the same age), so-called niche or affinity group retirement communities are composed of a subgroup of older people with shared characteristics who want to live near one another. These are purpose-built places for a targeted constituency, whether they be gay and lesbian baby boomers, retired union letter carriers, aging Asian-Americans, faith-based groups, artists, even recreational vehicle (RV) enthusiasts. Unlike most of the alternative models, these communities are usually created not by the residents themselves but by developers, both nonprofit and entrepreneurs. Some are affordable, others, pricey. Most are solely for independent "active" adults, but a few offer a continuum of health care services.

For example, Escapees CARE Center (CARE stands for Continuing Assistance for Retired Escapees) is not a nursing home for run-away convicts, but a nonprofit center for RV enthusiasts who are no longer able to hit the road. According to its website, CARE answers the question, "What happens to full-time RVers when they cannot take care of their own or their spouse's needs following an illness, injury, surgery, or the progression of a long-term health situation?"

The answer: come to Livingston, Texas, where they will find a "safe haven" at affordable prices, staffed by professionals. The goal is to allow people to continue to live in their RVs, in community with others, while getting the help they need. It promises, "The atmosphere at CARE is like an RV rally. It is nothing like a nursing home!" Pulling up your RV and taking advantage of such services as meals, transportation, housekeeping, and laundry costs $849 a month in 2012 (plus $36 a day to use the licensed adult day-care services on-site), compared to the national average for assisted living of $3550 a month.[1]

A 2010 AARP article noted, "The sense of community is the lifeline of CARE. Member donations make up about half of the nonprofit's operational budget, and volunteers help keep expenses low." The article tells of one woman who had moved there when her husband was dying of cancer and had found a genuine community who got her through the difficult ordeal. "If I had a bad day and things were rough, there was always someone to listen," she explained. "They were a tremendous support, and I knew I wasn't alone. . . . RVers are a breed of their own. They take care of each other. You make lifelong friends."[2]

Another emerging affinity community is aimed at those who practice Zen meditation. The San Francisco Zen Center hopes to develop a large parcel of land north of the city for a Zen-inspired continuing care retirement community. The idea was initially spawned by the Center's realization that they did not have enough rooms to house their aging monks, who are promised life-long housing and care after the age of seventy in return for twenty years or more of service to the community. "When we made that promise, we didn't think about where we're going to house people," said Susan O'Connell, president of the Center. "Our community is a very vibrant, ever-changing community—if we fill up all the rooms with a large portion of elders, there won't be enough room for people coming to train and participate."

According to Susan, the Center is one of the few intentional communities born in the 1960s and 1970s that not only still exists but is thriving. "We have figured out something about what makes community life work," she said. The Zen Center has a strong track record: it operates Greens, a successful vegetarian restaurant in San Francisco; manages an organic farm north of town; and runs a model hospice program.

Before proceeding with their plans to develop a retirement community, the Center conducted a marketing survey of its mailing list and other similar organizations. "We got a huge response, and it was very, very positive," said Susan. The idea is that the community will not be health-care-based, but lifestyle-based, with a large meditation hall, walking paths, and an organic farm or garden.

The Center partnered with Northern California Presbyterian Homes and Services to help develop the continuum of care they wish to provide. Both organizations have a vision that the "next paradigm for senior living" should be rooted in spirituality and community, said Susan.

The culture will not be a "dualistic" one dividing people into sick and healthy but rather will cultivate an attitude of "we're all in this together," she explained. Unlike many retirement communities that banish frailer people who use wheelchairs to their own separate wing, for example, everyone will mingle. "It's about presence and attention and listening," explained Susan. "It's the kind of shift that supports the caregiver more, and it allows the care receiver to not feel like they're 'less than.' From our first breath, we're all aging, we're all dying. It's a very Buddhist approach."

Based on the marketing survey, she anticipates that people from around the United States and beyond will want to move there. I asked if she would want to live there herself. "I'm building this for me," she laughed. "I'll be sixty-seven this year. I would definitely be a resident. I'm an elder here."

The Art of Aging

Another promising niche community is devoted to the arts and creativity. Research shows that the arts have the potential to contribute significantly to healthy aging. A 2012 study published in the *Journal of Aging and Health*, for example, identified "openness"—an integral part of being creative—as predictive of longer life. Openness and creativity have been found to reduce stress and contribute to cognitive health, among other benefits.[3]

A 2007 study in New York City, based on interviews with 213 artists aged sixty-two to ninety-seven, found that the respondents ranked high in life satisfaction and self-esteem, planned to keep working as an artist indefinitely, communicated daily or weekly with other artists, and went daily to the studio "even if it takes 1.5 hours to walk 2 blocks."

The researchers concluded: "Psychological models of 'successful aging' have highlighted evidence of positive personal growth, creativity, self-efficacy, autonomy, independence, effective coping strategies, sense of purpose, self-acceptance and self-worth. Artists, as our study makes abundantly clear, are engaged in all of these indicators."[4]

I called Gay Hanna, executive director of the National Center for Creative

Aging, who has spent her career immersed in the arts, older adults, and health and wellness. She reflected on why the arts could be a meaningful foundation for people wanting to live in a community as they grow old. "Art is spiritual, and it's community-building," she said. "It's also very physical and very mental. It has many, many entry points." In other words, the arts and creativity don't encompass only painting, sculpture, and dance, but also sewing, cooking, quilting, and gardening.

"Certainly the making of art allows one to express oneself and indeed allows us to tell our story," she added.

Telling our story is a fundamental developmental task of our older years. As the late Gene Cohen, MD, the pioneer of creativity and aging, explained, beginning at around age seventy people "feel more urgently the desire to find larger meaning in the story of their lives through a process of review, summarizing, and giving back . . . we begin to experience ourselves as 'keepers of the culture' and often want to contribute to others more of whatever wisdom and wealth we may have accumulated."[5] This desire takes many forms, such as memoir writing, organizing photographs and mementoes, oral history, and genealogy.

An example of the power of personal storytelling comes from Triangle Square in Hollywood, one of the first affordable housing complexes in the nation for gays and lesbians. It was built as a safe and secure place for people who may have faced a lifetime of discrimination. "We did a stage show with music of their personal stories of discovering their sexuality and it was fantastic," said Tim Carpenter, founding director of the nonprofit EngAGE. "These were people who had never told their story outside of their tribe, and it opened their eyes that people were fascinated with their journey. There is a sense of coming together about it."

A leader in the world of arts and aging, Tim Carpenter, like Brenda Eheart of Generations of Hope, is an Ashoka Fellow, recognized for creating innovative solutions to pressing social problems. He parleyed his love of the arts and creativity into EngAGE, which brings high quality artistic and learning programs and events to older adults who live in thirty low-income housing communities in Southern California, including a few that were established by Tim as Senior Artists Colonies.

Tim grew up near Yaddo, the famed artists colony in New York, which may have planted the seed for his vision. He also recalls hearing a talk given in the 1990s by Dr. Bill Thomas, the maverick geriatrician who has spent his career re-imagining eldercare. Bill Thomas, Tim recalled, spoke about a nursing home built in a neighborhood in San Diego made up of blue-collar and agricultural workers. The place had raised garden beds and a shop where re-tired guys from the trades could tinker. "That was the first thing that triggered in my mind—you could preplan the place based on the type of people who might live there," Tim said. "While I was sitting in that lecture, I wrote down senior artists colony. My wife thought the idea was cool, but the developers laughed."

He reflected on why he set out to create senior artists colonies in the Los Angeles area and beyond. "What's the ideal community? Part of it is living around people who you have empathy with," he said. "You can walk next door and know you have something in common with this person. You have a fused passion." In his case, he went on, if he were to live in a retirement community, "art is pretty cool and is a big part of my life. Most people who are close to me have some toe in that pool, whether they are artists or appreciators. I'd rather sit and talk about a movie or a novel or a piece of music than do just about anything." Being around others who feel the same way, he suggests, feeds his soul.

The bond does not have to be art, he added. His other fantasy is to create a retirement community of those linked by the desire for "wellness." He imag-ines avid bicyclists, hikers, organic gardeners, people who love to cook whole-some and delicious food, all living together in community. (In fact, he was speaking in Napa Valley and mentioned that dream, and afterward someone came up and immediately wanted to help him get it off the ground. It hasn't happened—yet.)

In 1999, Tim cold-called the city of Burbank and pitched the idea of a se-nior artists colony. Burbank, a city of 100,000 people in the middle of greater Los Angeles, is dominated by the entertainment industry, including such gi-ants as Disney, Warner Brothers, and Nickelodeon. Tim got lucky. The per-son who answered the phone that day, a project manager, immediately saw how a senior artists colony would be a good fit for their community. She was enthusiastic, assisting Tim in getting $3.5 million to subsidize the project. A for-profit developer, Meta Housing, was in charge of construction, and a management company called The Legacy operates the place, with EngAGE responsible for programming.

I met Tim and two artist-residents in the lobby of the Burbank Senior Art-ists Colony on a sunny September morning. Gregarious and funny, Tim is a tall, square-jawed man, with stylish heavy-rimmed glasses and sandy-red hair.

The four-story stucco building, painted cream, brown, and green, is at a busy intersection, with an inviting tree-canopied boulevard just outside the door. The building is surrounded by a flowerbed, lush with succulents and birds of paradise, and each apartment has either a balcony or a patio onto the courtyard. All 141 units are for those who can live independently, with 40 set aside as affordable housing.

Artistic works are everywhere: a large metal art sculpture hangs outside on an upper story while interior walls are covered with paintings and murals.

In the lobby, Tim introduced me to two of the most active artists, Suzanne Knode and Teddi Shattuck. I asked them what it's like to live in an artists colony. "It changes the whole way you live your life," said Suzanne. "Everything is different." She has opened herself to risk, trying things she'd never dreamed she'd do. "I have much more ambition now than I did when I was younger." She was working on her autobiography, told as a series of short stories.

Teddi, a hip-looking seventy-six-year-old who seemed to view the world through a sardonic lens, agreed. She had been a painter all her life (except when she was raising her four children—"oil painting and kids don't mix"), but she had never tried creative writing before. Since taking classes at the Artists Colony she's written a documentary and three plays, including *seniormismatch.com*, which was performed by the resident troupe. She had recently spent a month in Egypt, painting a mural on a school as a guest artist. While there, she wrote a play for the students in simple English. A former travel agent, she's been to over a hundred countries and was preparing to go to Surinam.

Suzanne's first class was a writing workshop led by Tim, and one of her first projects was a hilarious ten-minute screenplay called *Bandida*, the story of an older woman with a walker who takes a public bus to rob a liquor store. Suzanne ended up producing and directing a film of *Bandida*. *This American Life* even produced a segment on Suzanne making the film for their television series.[6]

Suzanne and Teddi told me of other residents who had blossomed through the arts. "A lady in her early nineties just wrote a book of poetry," Suzanne said.

"There's a gentleman named Buster who's lived here a couple years," she went on. "He writes all these little plays. One very funny one was of an elderly couple sharing a reminiscence. He thought they were talking about a bar mitzvah, and she thought it was a wedding. Buster wants to take it on the road to senior places."

Tim said he'd originally imagined the place being filled with established artists, but he's inspired by people "dusting off their dreams" and pursuing art for the first time as elders.

"You never know what the tide's going to bring in," Teddi opined of her fellow residents.

When I asked the average age of the residents, she wisecracked, "Old—too old. They should never have moved in in the first place." (In fact, the age range is late fifties to ninety-three, with an average age of late seventies.) Despite her tough exterior, Teddi devotes considerable time, energy, and talent to making the community a better place, as I was to learn.

Suzanne was also working on painting, in addition to writing and film. She showed us a portrait she had done of Sidney, a staffer who works for EngAGE. "There was a drum circle with a photo of Sidney dancing outside," Suzanne explained. She had been working on the picture for two months and had successfully captured the woman's face and hair, dreadlocks flying as she danced.

As we talked, I admired an art piece on the lobby wall. It was a wild, vibrant cutout on pressboard of a man and woman dancing. The colors were intense and the figures alive. The artist, I was told, was in his mid-eighties.

One of the Colony's success stories is a partnership between the elders and the at-risk teens who attend a high school next door. The kids and a few of the elders, in particular Teddi, work on a huge vegetable garden together. "The intergenerational program has been fabulous," said Tim. "We're now doing a graphic novels class with them. There's lots of collaboration with Disney and Nickelodeon. Warner Brothers did a workday in our garden."

Besides the artistic work, there's a raft of exercise classes and social activities. "We do have a real community here," said Suzanne. "Yesterday a resident's daughter had died, and there was a memorial service here for her. So many people were there to support Vonda." Suzanne said she has made a lot of good friends there, and that her oil painting class has grown especially close.

The community has a regular wine gathering they call "The Four O'Clock," which Teddi dubbed "The Unhappy Hour—everybody gets drunk and complains."

As we talked, residents came through the lobby, some headed outside with their small dogs trotting alongside. A sweet-looking woman walked by. Tim greeted her, but she didn't respond. She was deaf, it turned out. "She goes to everything," said Teddi. "Her son said if she hadn't moved here, she would have been dead by now."

Another woman had also been at death's door when she came there, but she lived much longer than anyone anticipated. In fact, Tim joked, "If there's an inheritance at play, you might not want your mother to move here."

But of course, there is no Fountain of Youth. Many people had died, including a wonderful sculptor. "Helen who played the Bandida lives with her daughter now," Suzanne said sadly. "She lost her memory. She had memorized the whole script."

Tim had another appointment, so he left me with Teddi and Suzanne for a tour. Two studios are open twenty-four hours a day. In one, a resident artist was teaching watercolor to other residents. When I told them I was writing a book about alternative ways people choose to live as we grow older, the teacher cracked, "I choose to be one of the idle rich, but it's just not working out." None of the students had ever painted before, and I was impressed with their images of landscapes and animals.

The other studio was filled with easels and oil paints. A few of Teddi's paintings leaned on easels and against cabinets. She typically spends her mornings there. In the afternoon, she works on her other passion, the intergenerational garden.

The monthly schedule of classes and activities was not like the usual retirement community—and one of the few places I've been that doesn't list Bingo. Among the offerings: Poetry Tool Box, Colony Chorus, Acting, Drum Circle, Philosophy, Theater, Mardi Gras–Mask Making, Healthy Eating, Anti-Aging Exercise, Yoga, Zumba, and Meditation. A small library overlooks the street, and a large poster advertising the latest performance by the Burbank Senior Artists Colony Players was propped on an easel.

The huge patio, unfortunately, is not used much, they told me, despite having loads of inviting tables with umbrellas, a stone pool with a sculpture of frogs floating on their backs on lily pads, and a barbeque grill. Neither is the room with a pool table. There's a small swimming pool on the patio that Teddi called "a hot tub on steroids."

Near the patio is the theater, with a stage and seating for forty. Every couple of months the residents put on an original play before an audience made up of other residents, family, friends, and people from the community. Teddi is also active in the theater group. She joked about people coming late to rehearsal, only to realize they'd forgotten their glasses. "Most people want to be participants," she said. "They don't care about the end result." The theater is also used by professional troupes.

The patio overlooks the Burbank School and the large garden with peaches, apples, raspberries, pomegranates, lemons, and blood oranges. "We introduce the kids to vegetables," said Teddi. "Many of them have never eaten vegetables. I cook with the kids—we've made fried green tomatoes, squash casserole. One boy said, 'I don't like that,' and then ate three helpings."

In addition to the garden, Colony residents have worked with the students on producing a clay animation film, "Unless You've Walked in My Shoes," written by a Latino student and filmed on location in city ballparks. The students did all the work, including learning how to edit, with the elders as mentors.

Teddi offered to show me her apartment. All the apartments are accessible, small but well-designed. Teddi's was crowded with an amazing conglomeration of stuff—acrylics tubes and paintbrushes on the kitchen counter, paintings packed on the wall, snapshots of her world travels, and unique wooden furniture that she had made. A guitar leaned on the couch. "I taught myself," she said casually—another shared project with the students. The Colony managed to get several guitars donated for this purpose.

"This place seems like it would fall apart without you," I observed. She shrugged. "A lot wouldn't get done," she said simply.

She and Suzanne expressed disappointment that more of the residents are not involved in the arts—perhaps twenty-five actively participate. Because of the recession, it had been hard to keep the apartments full, and they felt that many residents have moved in for the reasonable rents, rather than to explore their creativity.

Later, I asked Tim about the small number of participants, and he disagreed that there were so few. Some lifelong artists who live there prefer the solitude of working on their creative pursuits and are not joiners, he maintains. That said,

> We're always trying to find ways to get people as involved as they want. Someone a long time ago told me about senior programming—don't make them feel like they have to go to camp. Don't treat these people like they're thirteen-year-olds who have never been to a party before. I have to constantly remind myself they've been around the block a lot more than I have. They know how to live their life. We're just trying to make it a little better.
>
> People gather for conversation, not to be engaged in the programs. Things change. I've been doing this for fifteen years now. We've kept a lot and thrown away a lot—we've tried everything under the sun, short of hang gliding and things the developers wouldn't want us doing for insurance purposes. The concept is, make sure the place is cool, do as much as you can to promote the stories of the people who are doing it, make sure there's a lot going on. Use peer leadership, rather than someone like Tim Carpenter—people like Suzanne who wasn't an artist at all when she moved there. It's the idea of promoting through culminating events and creating reasons for people to get together and developing leaders in the community.

He is confident enough in the Senior Artists Colony model that he and Meta Housing were putting the finishing touches on two more: NOHO Senior Arts Colony in North Hollywood and Long Beach Senior Arts Colony.

NOHO has a seventy-eight-seat theater, home to the professional Road Theatre Company. Impressively, Long Beach's two hundred units are all designated as affordable housing. "The artistic spaces in the Long Beach project are really huge—a huge art studio, big gallery space, big media lab to do video, sound, and photo," said Tim. "It's a much larger building than the other two." There is also a nearby school, offering potential for intergenerational programming, and EngAGE is exploring a relationship with a dance company—a swap of space in exchange for dance programs for residents.

To ensure a critical mass of artists among the residents, the two new buildings have a new screening process for applicants. Artists will get a preference, and a panel will choose who is likely to make the most of the opportunity to live there. But even for those older people who have not been artists earlier in life, Tim added, "There's a pre-seeded, inherent promise. It's seeded in their head that they would want to go to a place like this. It isn't just because it's a nice location and I can afford to live there—at least that's the goal, and so far we've seen that work. A lot of people who end up living in these communities want to continue to practice the way they already live, or they want to change what they're doing. That's the only way to engage in community in a healthful way."

The primary question for any senior artists colony, he said, is, "How do we change the crucible within which this stuff takes place—where you create physical amenities with studios, and theaters, and media labs, and all the right spaces that match to this, and have intellectual amenities like classes, and reasons to get people to go downstairs and do something *real?* When you get professional artists in a place and you get persons to engage in something of a higher order, we see that people's lives change."

Nalcrest: "A Retirement That's Union-Made"

In Central Florida, amid alligator-filled lagoons, Spanish moss–draped live oaks, and orange groves, lies a unique and affordable community comprised of retired postal workers. All are members of their union, the National Association of Letter Carriers. Called Nalcrest, the community was envisioned by the late union president William Doherty as an affordable home in a warm climate for well-deserving workers who had spent their lives trudging through sleet and snow.

A team from the union scouted property and purchased a 150-acre parcel next to a large lake. They created two large lagoons, and purchased an adjoining 150 acres, which they keep undeveloped. Buildings were constructed with money from both the union and the US Department of Housing and Urban Development (HUD), which supports affordable housing.

"It was one of my husband's lifelong dreams to come here," said Janet, widow of a letter carrier who hopes to live at Nalcrest the rest of her life. "He hated the weather in Massachusetts and all the snow shoveling. We came to visit one year and moved the following year."

Unlike many retirement communities that are drawing an older crowd, Nalcrest residents often arrive as soon as they retire. With the union benefits, this can be as young as fifty-five, as with new arrival Bruce who had moved there from Honolulu. "It's a lot cheaper to be retired in Florida than it would be in Hawaii," he said. "Financially this was the best way for me to retire."

Indeed, one of the most impressive aspects of life at Nalcrest is its affordability—rents range from $395 for an efficiency to $520 a month for a two-bedroom apartment, including everything but the electric bill and phone.

As it prepared to celebrate its fiftieth anniversary, Nalcrest seemed to be thriving. Of the five hundred rental units, an average of 10 percent were vacant, mostly due to people passing away or moving because of frailty. In 2013 twenty veterans of World War II still lived at Nalcrest. Most residents are snowbirds, with only one hundred living there year-round.

Gary, sixty-one, and his wife moved there two years after he retired. Gary had visited Nalcrest when the union held a national conference in Orlando. "Several of us came down and said, 'Hey, this may be the place,'" he said. He likes that people come from almost every state to live there, yet they all share the bond of being "in the letter carrier family," as he put it. Like Janet, he plans to be there the rest of his life.

He ticked off the amenities Nalcrest offers: "We have our own post office, our own restaurant, a barber and beauty shop, Laundromat, chapel, fire station. They are just finishing renovation of the fifty-year-old swimming pool. The trustees added WIFI to the general community town center." The Doherty auditorium holds five hundred seats, and outside groups come to speak. They also have two tennis courts, bocce, basketball, and "an abundance of pinochle, poker, and canasta. You have so much here, you don't want to leave," he said.

They enjoy the natural landscape of Old Florida. "There's a brand new dock being built and abundant fishing. You can go picnicking and we have five grills out on the site by the big lake. You can watch sunrise and sunset, eagles, armadillos, and of course alligators. We have a new eagle family, with two hatchlings. We have deer, we have a panther. [I'm impressed. Florida panthers are endangered.] The nearest stores are ten miles west. We're out in the woods, and we love it."

Janet believes that living at Nalcrest "adds ten years to your life." While that sounds like hyperbole, the community can point to many features that may well contribute to residents' physical and mental well-being.

For one, the national union has won them outstanding benefits. "Most if not all residents here have a very quality type health insurance that's provided by our own union, in addition to some who are on Medicare," explained Matty Rose, a national trustee for the union who helps oversee Nalcrest. "When you can live very conservatively on a low amount, you don't have to be stressed out concerning the economy going up or down, you know what your pension is, and you know what your expenses are. You have a lot of stress taken off your shoulders. I'm no doctor, but when someone has peace of mind like that, I would think that plays significantly on their life."

Beyond the economic security, said others, is the strong sense of purpose and community that they share. Bruce, the "baby" of the group, heads up the Community Emergency Response Team, which serves not only Nalcrest but the nearby area. Residents organize food drives, raise funds for the Alzheimer's and Muscular Dystrophy Associations, and collect Toys for Tots for the Marine Corps. "We don't only take care of our own here," said Gary. "We take care of surrounding communities."

He agreed with Janet's assertion of a ten-year longevity benefit from being active. "On our softball field, Monday, Wednesday, and Friday, you see people from ages fifty-five to eighty-five or ninety. The older one hits, the younger one runs for him," he said. "You need to get out and smell the roses."

They are also politically active, which they view as part of being good union members. They regularly cover city and state legislative sessions and conduct grassroots lobbying campaigns on behalf of issues of concern to active and retired letter carriers. "You have to realize even though we're retired, we're still union, fighting for continuation of six-day delivery," Gary said, of the Postal Service proposal to eliminate mail delivery on Saturdays. "Here at Nalcrest, we have representation at the county seat, and twice a month we make county commissioner meetings." Among the other activities, the residents band together to write letters and do phone banking on legislative issues important to them.

"The eclectic makeup of Nalcrest represents the makeup [of the union]," said Matty Rose. "All colors and faiths and national origins, we all live together and get together, just like we all worked together. Whether you have a physical disability or are black or white or Asian or Hispanic, if you believe in God or don't believe in God, everybody here is in community. Not to say that every single resident likes another resident but we all live together in harmony."

Janet gave an example of what that social support has meant for her. "I tripped and fell during the summer and broke my shoulder," she said. "Gary and his wife Karen took care of me for three weeks while my arm was in a sling, feeding me and cutting up my food for me. We kind of look out for each other."

What about when people can no longer drive, I wonder. After all, they are out in the woods, some ten miles from stores and a hospital.

"This is where neighbors and residents come in," said Matty. "They help out and transport them to the grocery store. We do have a couple residents that provide some type of car service for a nominal amount, for doctor visits, or take them to the airport in Orlando. So there's all types of accommodations to get people into town for whatever reason they want to go." They are also petitioning the Polk County Commission to have at least some bus service to Nalcrest.

Their shared work history, he added, "absolutely creates a bond. This is probably the most unique benefit that any union offers for their membership," he said. "Unions offer pensions and discount programs but to have a community like this, at such a low price, for union members to take advantage of—I think we're very unique."

A Cautionary Tale

As I looked for niche communities to visit, I found one that advertised as by and for gay people. Its website promised a friendly community, lots of things to do, activities in the surrounding area, beautiful scenery, and reasonable rent. After some difficulty getting a response to calls and emails (that perhaps should have been a sign), I finally spoke to the man in charge who told me he would not be available when I came but that residents would be happy to talk to me.

Were they ever—but not in the way that any owner would want. When I arrived, my first interview was with someone I'll call Bruce. He was a short fellow in his late sixties, who looked like an average Joe. He still worked full-time as a caregiver for a person with mental disabilities. We sat in the empty community dining room, near a counter with a coffeemaker that did not appear to have been used recently. I began with my spiel that I was working on a book that looks at alternative ways people are choosing to live as they grow older.

He stopped me. "I have to quibble with the word 'choosing,'" he said. Somewhat startled, I asked him to elaborate. I wondered if he thought I meant he was "choosing" to be gay. But no, that wasn't it.

The problem was that he felt stuck. Having never had the opportunity to live in a gay community before, he had been looking forward to moving there. "I was astounded to find a place online that was a gay-friendly establishment for seniors," he said. "I've been out [as a gay person] for forty-five years and mostly lived in the heterosexual community." When he came to visit, he felt really catered to. "But you move here," he said, "and it's really oppressive."

What he and others discovered was an owner (himself gay) with serious issues, who ran the place more like a cranky tyrant than a friendly inn-keeper.

I asked Bruce if he had heard about any discrimination against gay people who live in traditional retirement communities. He offered the example of a Jewish man who, when he needed more services, had left their community and moved to a Jewish continuing care community. "They asked him to leave when they learned he was gay," according to Bruce.

Bruce himself had had a stroke in 2008. "It took a lot of the vibrance out of me," he said. "My energy level is half of what it was. I looked at a few places to live. I looked at traditional retirement communities—one was just studio apartments. One I really considered was predominantly Russians and Ukrainians—too conservative." He could have remained in a straight community. "When you pass all of your life, it's easy to do. And I have a lot of friends outside of the gay community. At sixty-seven I'm not exactly bringing home throngs of people. Part of me wants to, but part of me can't," he joked of his romantic life. "I'm at the point where I would like things to be simple."

He had hoped to find that when he moved. He had read in a news article that the owner promised residents would feel "safe and secure." But instead, the environment was fraught.

One of many examples he gave of the owner's peculiar behavior was a time when the WIFI was down, so that Bruce could not use the Internet. When he went to tell the owner, he flew into a rage. "He perceives everything as confrontation," Bruce said.

Activities that were promised do not occur. The community dining room was only used if one of the men bought pizza to share (all the residents are men but one).

Bruce led me down the hall to show me his modest apartment. Along the way, he pointed to the décor. "All the guys complain it looks like a nursing home for little old ladies," he said. He was right. As someone who has written about nursing homes, I found the place felt awfully familiar. There was flowered wallpaper, plastic flowers, and fussy figurines on side tables—reflecting the building's former life as an assisted living center, as it turns out. "We're *gay* people," he said with frustrated humor. "We like good design and cool things."

In his apartment, he had a collection of religious art, representing his Greek Orthodox background. Like all the apartments, he had only a kitchenette with microwave and small refrigerator—so cooking was not an option. He found that the low rent was undercut as he spent more on eating out than he would with a full kitchen.

We went out a side door to a stoop where a few men were chewing the fat and smoking. They had informally adopted a neighborhood cat that trotted over to say hello and nibble some food the men put out. The grounds bordered a day care center, and the men were enjoying watching youngsters in the playground.

"We'd like to be more a part of the community," said Bruce. But again, the owner made it difficult. One of the residents invited his church group to come there for Bible study. The owner glowered at them so much, I was told, that the group declined to return.

Another resident and clearly a leader of the pack I'll call David. A handsome man, with a full head of wavy blond hair and a sardonic wit, David, seventy, had lost much of his savings caring for his life partner of forty-two years, "Scott," who had died a few years earlier. We began our conversation in his apartment, where he showed me photos of Scott, whom he clearly missed deeply. Scott had had heart disease and died at seventy-four. They had moved to Florida from San Francisco, so that Scott's family could help care for him. "When he died, I didn't know what to do," said David. "I had lost contact with friends. I searched for places on the web. When I found this one, I thought I'd have instant friends and it would be a comfortable place I could settle down in. And I do feel comfortable because of the people—I just didn't know I'd run into a lunatic landlord."

Like Bruce, David felt trapped by his lack of financial resources. "At our age, you're limited on income. You can't just say I'm out of here," he said.

My last interview was with a gentle soul, "Charles." Charles told me he is a cross dresser who had lived almost his entire life closeted in the Bible belt of Florida. The political choices there, he smiled, were "Republican or Tea Party." "I wanted the companionship of being able to talk with people of similar inclination," he said. Not only was he tired of hiding his identity, but he wanted to find a place with more services, such as public transportation. "I did research on the Internet and this was the only [gay community] that was affordable," he said.

He tried to do due diligence and made several visits. When he first moved there, the place had dining service and a good manager. The manager used to organize activities and outings, such as participating in the local gay pride march or AIDS walks. They would go on hikes and eat together at local restaurants. But the manager left and was not replaced, as a cost-cutting measure, according to Charles. Dining services also ended.

As I looked around the empty and now forlorn seeming dining room, I asked him what a typical day was like. He gets up and goes out—perhaps to the library or on an errand. He eats lunch and takes a nap. He works out in the small gym in the building. "I've been living on bacon and tomato sandwiches," he said, smiling. He and David planted a garden, which he enjoys. "I like to see things grow," he said. "I grew up on a farm."

"I get along good with everybody," he said.

I asked if he had any advice for someone looking for a community, given what happened to him. "I checked it out over a period of time, but even doing so, you can't foresee what the future will bring," he said. "My advice to people would be to obtain as much flexibility as they can because you never know what life will bring."

I left there feeling dispirited. Unless the owner decided to sell, it seems like the community would not survive. Only about one-third of the units were rented, and the owner did little to attract new people. Bruce and David told me they felt guilty because their last best hope was to get a critical mass of newcomers who would work with them to force some good changes—stage a coup of sorts. But to get new people, they had to lie about the dismal state of affairs. They had managed to convince one lesbian to come, and she apparently felt deceived, once she'd moved there and saw how unhappy a place it was.

Why do I share this story? The lesson I drew was that having as much control as possible over our living situation is critically important. And in fact, it helps explain why so many people want to age in place—perhaps as much as having their familiar surroundings is knowing they have control.

Gay Retirement Living

As the previous example suggests, one group with cause for particular concern about how they will live as they grow older is lesbian, gay, bisexual, and transgender adults. Research is limited, but an estimated two to three million older LGBT adults live in the United States. According to Caring and Aging with Pride, the first national federally-funded project to explore LGBT aging and health, significant disparities exist between this population and the aging population generally. Surveys of 2,560 LGBT people aged fifty to ninety-five found that respondents were at greater risk of disability, physical and mental distress, victimization, discrimination, and lack of access to supportive aging and health services.[7]

When asked about needed services, respondents ranked housing first, followed by transportation, legal services, social events, and support groups.[8] More than half reported being discriminated against in employment and housing. Five percent had been unable to move to the neighborhood they wished "as a result of their actual or perceived sexual orientation or gender identity."[9]

LGBT elders are less likely to have children or other family members to turn to for assistance. As a sixty-six-year-old lesbian said in the survey, "Isolation, finding friend support, caregiving, and health are the biggest issues older gay persons face. Who will be there for us, who will help care for us without judgment?"

A 2010 survey on the experience of LGBT elders in long-term care settings was also troubling. Respondents included gay people themselves, as well as family members, friends, and providers of legal and social services. Only 22 percent of LGBT respondents thought they could be open if they moved to a long-term care facility; the non-LGBT respondents were even more pessimistic, with only 16 percent saying long-term care residents could be out of the closet. Among the concerns the survey revealed: abuse or neglect by staff, isolation from other residents, and discrimination by both residents and staff. Respondents reported verbal or physical harassment from other residents and from staff, refused admission or sudden discharge, restriction of visitors, and staff refusing to accept power of attorney from the resident's partner.[10]

"I would say of the many complex decisions you're making [as an older adult], one of them shouldn't be am I going to be discriminated against or am I going to feel safe here, and unfortunately for many LGBT adults it is," said Serena Worthington, director of Community Advocacy and Capacity Building for SAGE (Services and Advocacy for Gay, Lesbian, Bisexual & Transgender Adults). "I would add that affordability is a very big concern." She points out that many retirement programs and policies favor married couples.

Worthington, who worked in a nursing home for four years, said that today's oldest heterosexual people have lived through much upheaval in society, including the civil rights movement. "I don't think it's impossible that people change," she said. "It's a generation, while capable of great transformation, [that] also has supported discrimination against LGBT people. Are they going to be warm and fuzzy? Is this going to be an environment where you'll feel comfortable as an out lesbian couple? Probably not. I'm sure there are some progressive communities, but there are many places where that couldn't happen."

Progress has been made, at least in some areas, regarding housing discrimination. According to Lambda Legal, as of December 2012 sixteen states and the District of Columbia, as well as one hundred municipalities, had enacted laws banning discrimination based on sexual orientation and gender identity and expression. Another five states ban discrimination based on sexual orientation (without addressing gender identity and expression). The US Fair Housing Act and the Nursing Home Reform Act also offer LGBT people some legal protection against discrimination. Still, the majority of states do not ban discrimination based on sexual orientation.

Despite the extra burdens faced by many LGBT elders, the picture is not grim by any means for many others, perhaps even the majority. Many have "chosen family" rather than blood kin for support and companionship. In a 2010 study by Metlife Mature Market Institute, LGBT respondents by significant margins were more likely to turn to close friends for support, compared to a general population comparison group, including to confide in, for help with errands, for support and encouragement, in an emergency, and for advice.[11]

While some express interest in living in a gay retirement community, Worthington said that others, especially younger and more affluent people, would prefer living in a mixed community. "They like the vibrancy of multiple ages and different kinds of people," she said. "I do think actually—not in older adult settings, but generally—LGBT people are experiencing a kind of reprieve from discrimination in some settings so we're more assimilated and feel less need for set-aside places. There are hardly any lesbian bars anymore, because there doesn't need to be. Lesbians can go to any bar, or I could live anywhere."

At the same time, she said, "There is definitely a real drive in humans for affinity. . . . In a perfect world where there wasn't discrimination, I think people might make choices based on affinity in all kinds of ways."

In response to both perceived discrimination and the desire for living with like-minded folks, a handful of gay retirement communities have emerged. Some, like Triangle Square in Hollywood, are designated as affordable housing. Other affordable communities include 55 Laguna in San Francisco, 3600 North Halsted in Chicago, Spirit on Lake in Minneapolis, and John C. Anderson Apartments in Philadelphia.

Others are more upscale, such as Fountaingrove Lodge in Santa Clara, California; BOOM in Palm Springs; The Palms of Manasota in Palmetto, Florida; and Carefree Cove in Boone, North Carolina. Several others never got off the ground or went bankrupt, victims of the recession and collapse of the housing market.

One that is off to a good start is Birds of a Feather, outside Pecos, New Mexico. "The seed got planted many years ago," said Bonnie McGowan, sixty-three, the developer and first resident of the community. "When I was in my thirties, everyone was still pretty closeted. There was a big concern about when we age, where will we go? Will we be separated from our partners? It was almost universal that people would be at a party and start talking about what are we going to do when we get older."

Bonnie has a strong family background in real estate development and construction. She went on to become a highly successful partner in a Minneapolis brokerage firm. Her experience gave her the confidence to develop a community. "All my customers were institutional clients, so I knew how to deal with banks, and I wasn't intimidated by the process of undertaking a pretty large investment risk," she said. "So I decided to pursue the idea of creating this community."

She began in the mid-1990s by conducting an informal online survey to gauge interest among lesbians and gays. She got a strong response from people saying they would be interested in living in such a community. She also solicited respondents' views on where they would like a community to be. She expected that people would say Florida, but instead the top choices were California, Arizona, and New Mexico. With California being expensive and Arizona scorchingly hot in summer, she said, New Mexico seemed the best choice. Having vacationed in Santa Fe, Bonnie decided to focus her search there. It took her two years to find the right piece of property, a 160-acre parcel surrounded by National Forest with a 360-degree view of the mountains.

To Bonnie, a nature lover and environmentalist, the setting was a dream come true. As she describes it on the website: "The Pecos Wilderness is a vast wonderland of fir and aspen groves, emerald lakes, and alpine meadows with waves of grass and purple irises, all framed by the Sangre de Cristo Mountains."[12]

She completed the purchase in 1999 but that was just the first step. "It's been a long and difficult journey," she said.

Some local folks had used the land for cattle grazing, and they fought her construction permit. Although many observers assumed that opponents were resistant because it was a gay community, she doesn't think so. "I had three strikes against me: I was a woman, I was from back East, and I was an Anglo," she said. Her case went to the New Mexico Supreme Court, where she won. "I'm stubborn. It took its toll as far as time and money, but I was still committed to doing the project."

Because of the delays, she did not break ground until 2004. She quickly sold all eighteen building lots. She built her own home on one, and over the next few years seven more adobe homes were completed. Once the recession hit, no new construction went on, but now four more are in the planning stages. She also received permission for eighteen additional building lots. She is marketing the community again and has been "bombarded" with emails of interest. Many people who contact her, though, cannot afford the $300,000 to $600,000 the homes cost.

She used much of her retirement savings to get the project off the ground and has yet to see a profit, although she is confident she will do fine financially. "I live here," she said. "I'm not a typical developer. I'm living a dream."

I asked her if gay retirement communities were mostly a reaction to discrimination, or were they instead a longing to settle "with your tribe." Bonnie responded that she's frequently asked in an era of marriage equality and other progress toward civil rights for gays if there is really a need for a separate community. While she welcomes how much progress has been made, she said, "Our country is so divided right now. It's very clear in all the elections—half are very conservative and do not support equality for gays. I always said until I can walk down the street of any community in the country holding my partner's hand, there is a need for a place for us, and a safe place." Indeed when she first conducted her marketing surveys, safety was the number one concern motivating people.

But it's also true, she said, that she and her neighbors were drawn to live near people with similar life experiences and views, just like others in any niche community. "People like to be with people who have like minds and like interests," she said. "All of us in that age range have experienced a lot of similar life experiences and so most of the people in the community are pretty liberal. They are intelligent, they've been successful, they're very active, they like to travel, go golfing, and do volunteer work." Residents of Birds of a Feather quickly became immersed in the life of the greater Pecos community, including running the food bank, being involved in Big Brothers and Sisters, and serving on the board of the Pecos Medical Center. Bonnie volunteers at the Wildlife Center. Several residents helped organize the Medical Center's annual fundraiser, called the "Pecos Pony Up," which included an auction and dinner dance. "Gays and lesbians were dancing with each other and with the locals," she said. It was a huge success, raising a record amount.

Michael, who lives at Birds with his partner of thirty-eight years, David, said he would not likely move to a traditional retirement community. "Not unless I knew somebody that could give me some insight," he said. "I don't want to move into a community where I'm surrounded by straight people who may be homophobic or condemning of that lifestyle where I might not feel comfortable."

Michael and David are both from the Santa Fe area originally but had been living for many years in Las Vegas. When they heard about Birds and the chance to be near their families again, they immediately checked it out and quickly made up their minds to build a home there.

Here, said Michael, he and David have found "framily"—friends as close as family members. They spend considerable time with their neighbors, drinking morning coffee, hiking, golfing, going to movies, even traveling to Europe and Mexico together.

"It's a wonderful place to retire," Michael said. "It's truly enjoyable. I'm really very happy."

He is on the board of the Medical Center and does other volunteer work. I asked if he and David felt accepted by the wider community.

"Absolutely," he said. "I went to Santa Fe High, and we used to have this rivalry with Pecos. Whenever we'd come up here, we were constantly in fights. When you talked about gay issues, there were a lot of problems in this rural community. They were very, very nonaccepting. When we got back here, it seemed the mindset had changed entirely. People were so very friendly. People would treat us nice and warm and extend a lot of hospitality to us. As we were building in this community, we tried to use local builders, and they were all nice and friendly. I can't imagine a better place and we intend to stay here as long as we can."

Ellen, who heads the homeowner's association and at sixty-four is the oldest of the community, never imagined she'd find such a place to live. "I never thought I'd live with a community," she reflected. "When I was younger being gay wasn't exactly an easy thing. The concept of many gay people gathered together in a single location wasn't within my knowledge or expectation. As I got older and thought about retiring, it became evident to me that I couldn't survive alone or even with a partner out in the middle of nowhere.

"This was the next best alternative. I live in the forest, I can hike, my dogs can run loose, and yet I'm surrounded by people who are not only like-minded in terms of how I feel about nature but are equally like-minded about community and caring for each other. Aside from being kind and generous, they're incredibly bright and challenging."

She, her partner, and another resident have taken up saxophone lessons. With other neighbors she walks the dogs and exercises. Holidays are usually spent together in community.

As we talked on the phone, she told me that she was looking out her window at a dozen wild turkeys. In the summer, she said, hundreds of humming-birds arrive, so many that their thrumming wakes her up in the morning.

Ellen said she has thought about what will happen as she grows older. Both her parents had dementia, and she worries about what her own future might hold. She jokes that maybe, "I won't know who I am but I can push the wheel-chairs for those who can't walk." The homes have all been built as single-story, with handrails in the tub and other design features with frailty in mind. She intends to live to be a healthy one hundred-year-old, she said, staying in the community until the end.

I asked Bonnie if she thought she was the leading edge of a trend, or would gay retirement communities remain just a few scattered outposts. "The concept is so new, and so few have been successful," she said. "It will change as the economy strengthens and more baby boomers age, and there's more demand. Anybody older than me has been more closeted than my genera-tion. I don't get many over age sixty-five that don't have that fear of living in a gay-identified community. There are exceptions, trailblazers, who are not as fearful. As for people younger than me, I've heard, well it's so much easier for people who are younger that there's no need for this community."

She disagrees. "There is still bullying of teenagers. They kill themselves," she said. "I hope things change for younger people and I hope at some point there's no longer a need for this kind of community for people to feel safe about who they are, but even if we get to that point, I still see a need for a place for people of like minds and like interests."

CHAPTER 10

Housesharing

Finding Companionship
with Friends—or Strangers

Lindsay, a market researcher for builders and developers, was unhappy with her boss and her hour-long commute each way to work. She was only fifty-nine, but she realized that she was in a position to retire—far earlier than she'd ever imagined. "I knew it meant I wouldn't have a lot of money, but I could get by," she said. To avoid dipping into her savings, she rented out her basement and other rooms in her large home in the Cleveland Park neighborhood of Washington, DC.

At the same time, her friend of twenty-five years, Sandy, also had a large home and was hoping to cut expenses. After considerable discussion, the two decided to join forces.

Lindsay and Sandy are among a growing number of adults sharing a household. For most people, housesharing is motivated by the need to live more cheaply. That was demonstrated by a big jump in shared households that took place during the recession: from 19.7 million to 22 million, an 11.4 percent increase, from 2007 to 2010.[1] The study found that people with lower incomes were more likely to be sharing homes.

Of those sharing a home, more than three million adults were sixty-five and over in 2010. (In the Census definition, shared households are those with more than one adult over eighteen, not in school, and not spouses or cohabiting partners of the householder, thus it includes both related and unrelated adults.) Although most shared households are made up of family members (see next chapter), more than six million of the twenty-two million adults who lived together in 2010 were not related.

"It's important to think about homesharing as extremely flexible and customizable," said Kirby Dunn, executive director of HomeShare Vermont. "Shared housing can be a component of Villages and NORCs, it can be a housing type and a tool that works with other community models, and a stand-alone approach that works well for independent living or added services. As opposed to traditional senior housing or a stand-alone entity, it's really flexible."

Oz Ragland, a national leader of the cohousing movement, is a big believer in housesharing. "I find [the increase in people sharing houses] really exciting," he said. Both cohousing and housesharing offer people a way to stay closely connected to others and avoid isolation and loneliness. Oz is developing a handbook aimed at encouraging people to live together by providing real-world examples, resources, and practical tools.

After living for years in Songaia Cohousing near Seattle and worrying about the community's budget, he and his wife, in their fifties, decided it was time for a simpler living arrangement. They, along with a seventy-four-year-old couple and a twenty-nine-year-old single man, decided to move together into a roomy house on 1.3 acres adjoining Songaia. The house is owned by a small company they created, made up of five families, two who live there and three who live at Songaia. Oz and his housesharers pay rent to the company. "That has tax advantages," he said. "I'm a renter from that company. The rent can include anything we want. We, for example, want the rent to cover our Internet. Our utilities are all bundled into our rent, and that's a business expense to the company."

They find they need few rules to govern the household but base their actions on common sense and respect for the others. For example, they considered whether to have "quiet hours" at night. "We talked about it, and we realized it's kind of silly," he said. "What is the rule? We wouldn't make noise after ten o'clock? We know that would bother some of the people, so we wouldn't do it. We've tested how loud to have the television for example. The house is all hardwood and it echoes, unfortunately—that's one of the things that you don't want in a shared household."

Oz is motivated more by the close connections than by the financial benefits. "Here, we have this long history," he said. "Mostly what we have is understanding of each other's needs, and we respect and care for each other."

⊘⊘⊙

In their book, *My House, Our House*, the three author-friends, Louise, Jean, and Karen, tell the story of buying a house together outside Pittsburgh in 2004, when they were in their fifties. Calling it a cooperative household, which they named Birchwood (or Old Biddies Commune as they joke), they share practical advice and lessons learned from the experience. The experiment is working so well that they now can't imagine living alone.

For one, they find the financial savings are significant. They live in a larger, nicer home than any of them had before, yet their expenses from sharing utilities and maintenance make it more affordable. They all pitch in and do their fair share, although that does not mean every task is shared equally—one likes gardening while another tackles wiring the outdoor lighting. Two enjoy cooking, the other doing dishes.

As they planned for this big life change, they sensibly made a list of worst-case scenarios and discussed with an attorney how they would handle them. The list included such things as "two people deciding that the third was not working out and seeking to have that person leave," "the death of one or more of us," and "one person allowing strangers or relatives to move in without the consent of others." They hammered out in writing how each potential problem would be solved. For example, to protect the interests of all in case one of them dies, they each took out a small life insurance policy that named the others as beneficiaries. Each woman's heirs would still receive her share of home equity. They agreed to set limits on overnight guests to seven consecutive nights and twenty-one total days per year. In the case of "irreconcilable differences," they would retain a mediator, and if that failed, an arbitrator, to help them through it.

Jean's daughter, Maureen, wrote about how her mother's new living situation affected her. Like many adult children, she had always felt a sense of ownership and belonging in her mother's house—the last refuge for when things go wrong, or, as she put it, "Hotel Uh-Oh." But after her mother moved into her cooperative house, things weren't the same. When Maureen had a mini-crisis,

> I naturally assumed that I could stay at Mom's for a few weeks until I recovered from my drama at the time, but—gasp—I was declined! There was no clause for such an activity in Mom's residential agreement—this was no joke. This new house where my mother now lived was *not* my house.
>
> As time passed, however, I discovered that knocking before entering someone's living space, waiting to be invited to a meal before eating, and hanging one's jacket in the hall closet really wasn't so awful. In fact it's pretty reasonable. My visits to my mother's house are only slightly less indulgent than they were when I declared myself the co-owner of her things.[2]

Lindsay and Sandy

A strong sense of respect and caring led Lindsay to sell her house and move in with Sandy. Lindsay also wanted the financial benefits of housesharing. The move meant a significant change in lifestyle, especially for Lindsay, going from homeowner and landlord to tenant. Sandy already was renting out her large third floor, so initially Sandy told Lindsay she would have to make do with the guest room and den. One of Lindsay's friends cautioned her to not settle for too little. "She told me to negotiate the space so that I'm not living at the fringes but instead, that it becomes 'our' house." Lindsay felt there was a lot of "emotional wisdom" in her friend's advice and she asked Sandy for more space.

Sandy agreed that Lindsay could also include the living room as part of her space. It was seldom used. But then Sandy realized that meant getting rid of her own furniture that was in the room. "She had a meltdown. It was her grandmother's furniture—her grandmother was precious to her. She couldn't do it," said Lindsay. "I started looking at condos."

But in the end, she moved in. "In my mind, I didn't like the image of coming home to an empty apartment," she said. She believes it was the right decision. On a practical level, she was relieved to be out from under a big mortgage and high home maintenance costs. Perhaps more important, she is a gregarious and highly social person, and she appreciates Sandy's companionship.

As Sandy recalled it, nearly three years later, that moment of having to rearrange her downstairs was a particularly difficult one. Sandy had been a landlord for years. She had always drawn a bright line between her space and her tenants. They were to remain in their upstairs rented rooms, which included a microwave and small refrigerator. They could use the laundry room and the main kitchen—but only if Sandy wasn't there.

But with Lindsay, a friend who was to share the house, the expectations were quite a bit different. "I was not prepared," said Sandy. "I didn't know how hard it would be. My perception before was that it would not be all that intrusive. The emotional ramifications were a complete surprise to me. I had no idea how attached I was to the way my space looked and felt."

In fact, she said, "I felt pieces of the house weren't mine anymore. It's hard to say this—you picture yourself a flexible, mature adult, and then I discovered my house was part of my identity. What I was reading in Lindsay's changing things was that it wasn't good enough."

I asked Sandy what made her persevere, given the burden that she felt. "You mean what are the positives?" she responded. Without hesitation, she ticked them off: "Safety, companionship, help, friendship, it's enjoyable. . . . This one is hard to talk about, but Lindsay brings something to my life that I need, even though it's hard for me. I'm a low-energy introvert. I feel I need [her presence] to keep from being a lonely and alone old woman."

Lindsay reminded her friend that she also said she wanted to be kept flexible.

"I wanted to be stretched," Sandy agreed. "But I put it on the castor oil list. I had visions—you grow old, you close in, and I didn't want that."

Their commitment to their friendship helped them overcome their many differences. For example, Sandy liked to keep the temperature at 72°, winter and summer. "I think that's immoral!" said Lindsay of what she sees as extravagant and wasteful energy use. They now compromise and keep the thermostat at 68° in winter and 75° in summer. Kitchen space also had to be negotiated, with each using particular shelves in the refrigerator and pantry. Sandy's decorating choice runs to deep reds and blues, with solid furniture and collectibles like toaster racks and a Victrola. Lindsay has a spare aesthetic with a beach theme. At the same time, Sandy hates clutter and Lindsay is a sprawler.

Basically, Lindsay said, "I have more porous boundaries. Sandy will feel, 'that's mine—don't dare use it unless you ask.' I have to be careful not to cross her boundaries."

Once they made it through the transition period, it's been pretty smooth sailing. The two have worked out a daily rhythm that feels right. They cook and eat separately unless one invites the other to dine, usually about once a week. Yet they go out together frequently at night. "We've gotten closer through this process," said Lindsay. "I feel more sure about the close connection in this relationship. We reassure each other that problems are not a threat to our friendship."

They've also been creative about sharing finances and chores. Sandy was paying a lawn service—Lindsay likes yard work, so Sandy now pays her. Lindsay uses some of the money on landscaping that they both enjoy.

Nevertheless, they both realized that Lindsay's initial expectation that it was truly a shared household would not be met. The house is Sandy's, and while she does share much of the space, she is too attached to the house to see it as anyone's but her own. She does not allow Lindsay or any tenant to have overnight male guests, for example. "I don't like not being able to come down to breakfast in my skivvies," is how she puts it.

I asked them what their expectations are of each other. "I try to limit my expectations to what friends would do who did not live together," said Sandy. "If her car breaks down in the middle of the night, I'd expect Lindsay to call me. The difficulty is with the larger things—Lindsay's natural inclinations of generosity and nurturing are three times as large as mine. I've been conscious of trying not to take advantage of that."

Sandy asked Lindsay if she were surprised by Sandy's "stinginess."

Lindsay considered. "I thought by being generous, it would evoke a similar response from you," she said. "And it didn't."

While this may all sound like a difficult conversation—the stuff of a *Dr. Phil* or *Oprah* show—their revelations were constantly interrupted by laughter at each other and their ups and downs. I learned how deep their friendship was and how much they'd been through together. When Sandy's sister was dying of ovarian cancer, it was Lindsay, having just retired, who took care of her for three months. Sandy, who was not close to her sister, did not want to become involved in her care. "In my fashion I would have just hired somebody," she said. "It was Lindsay who pulled me kicking and screaming. She said, you need to do this for your peace of mind. It was a time when Lindsay and I were together a lot in emotional and stressful circumstances, and it led to an increase in intimacy and connection. I felt like she knew me for the ungenerous person I was."

Their main advice to anyone who is considering sharing a house: don't keep things locked up inside. If something is bugging you, talk about it. Otherwise blow-ups are inevitable. Writing down your understanding of how things will be, such as finances, is also important. Had they done that, they would have avoided the misunderstanding over whose house it ultimately was.

Whether they will live together forever is not clear. For now, the only reason they can think of for breaking up the household would be if either became a grandmother and wanted to move near family or if their health failed.

Later, Sandy said, "There's no question that the good outweighs the bad. Even when I was really resentful and stressed and really faced with the negatives, when it would have been so easy to say I give up—those words never came out of my mouth because the stuff on the other side was too compelling."

Robin and Nancy

Another creative way of living is to move in close proximity to friends without actually sharing the same space. When they were in their seventies, Nancy and Robin each got an apartment in the same rambling house in the Roland Park neighborhood of Baltimore. In another apartment lived a couple who also were good friends of the women.

Nancy, now eighty, said her friendship with Robin, who died in 2010, was unusually close. They initially were neighbors in the Bolton Hill section of Baltimore, meeting in 1980. They later became walking buddies as Robin was going through a painful divorce, and Nancy, a widow, was also extricating herself from a difficult romantic relationship. "We walked for two miles every day of the week," recalled Nancy. "Then we began traveling together."

As we talked, Nancy kept adding to the list of adventures she and Robin shared: traveling to Turkey, Spain, Portugal, Italy—twice, Vietnam and Cambodia, England, France, New Zealand, Croatia, Malta, and on and on. "Oh and we went down the Susquehanna (in Maryland) on a camping trip," and later, "How could I forget we went down the Colorado in a wooden dory?"

"We were very compatible," said Nancy. "She was the most amazing person I ever met. She never said a mean word about anyone. She was a wonderful, charming, elegant woman who had not had an easy life."

During one of their daily walks, Nancy told Robin about an article she'd read by a woman who had bought a big house with a few friends. Nancy and Robin daydreamed about doing the same thing. Robin was then living in the Roland Park neighborhood, known for its huge old houses with high ceilings, spacious dining rooms, many bedrooms, even music rooms, and large yards. Perhaps someday, they thought, they'd buy one of these and houseshare with friends. They imagined hiring a cook and "a lawn man." They discussed how expenses could be shared, and how carefully they would choose other housemates.

In the end, they made a different choice. Robin moved into one of the grand houses that had been converted into five apartments. Three years after settling in, she called Nancy. "The second floor is empty," she said. Nancy immediately moved in above her long-time friend.

They spent three happy years, each in her own apartment in the large house. "Robin would come up to my apartment in her pajamas and we'd have red wine and watch a movie together," Nancy said, smiling at the memory. They would often eat dinner together and help each other with chores. "I loved to garden and she was not a great gardener," Nancy said, so she helped Robin with weeding, mulching, and planting. Robin didn't mind driving and Nancy preferred organizing their trips and navigating. Robin didn't enjoy cooking, so Nancy would be more likely to invite her to a meal, or they would eat out together.

"We'd sit on her porch and talk sometimes. When we really bonded was when we were walking," Nancy said. "I shared things with her I'd never shared with anybody else, and she, the same."

Despite their closeness, they maintained boundaries. "Housesharing would have worked, but what we did was better," she said. "I was careful not to barge into her space if I went out to the garden. We honored each other's space."

It was at the end of yet another trip—this one down the Snake River in Idaho—when Robin told her dear friend that she had lymphoma. She had found out soon before the trip and almost didn't go, but didn't want to disappoint Nancy.

Robin was a fighter until the end. An avid tennis player, she kept it up even during cancer treatment. When she died in January 2010, Nancy said, "It was a terrible loss for me—like losing my husband."

She remained in her apartment for a while, but without Robin it wasn't the same. She moved to a continuing care retirement community, where her eighth floor corner apartment commands a breathtaking view of the city. She's glad to be there. I asked if she has the same sense of control and ownership as when she had her own apartment.

"They have very few rules and regulations here," she said. "I use the pool three times a week. They have good health care here. The staff is wonderful." She's made some good friends and appreciates the parties the management organizes, as well as impromptu cocktails in neighbors' apartments. But "there's not a man here I'd touch with a ten-foot-pole," she joked. And sometimes she tires of dining with so many others. "Sometimes you get sick and tired of everybody, so I bring my dinner up here," she said. "But it's a great way of meeting new people."

She likes living in an age-restricted community. There has been talk of bringing a nursery school to the campus, she said, "But most people don't want it—don't want the noise. If I wanted to be around children, there's a school right across the street where I could volunteer."

Still, if Robin hadn't died, Nancy would have preferred remaining in the apartment. "We thought we'd be there for the duration," she said.

Sharing a House with a Stranger

For those who have no best friend with whom they can live, housesharing is still an option. Across the nation, from Baltimore to Washington State, homeshare programs are cropping up as a way both to provide affordable housing and to help people age in place without being isolated. The National Shared Housing Resource Center (NSHRC), a loose-knit network, has identified some forty programs in eighteen states that offer matchmaking services for home providers and home seekers. In most cases, living with strangers is prompted by financial need on the part of both parties.

Housing is among the most pressing and expensive concerns of older people. According to a 2009 study by researchers at Brandeis University and Dēmos, a public policy organization, "High housing costs put 45 percent of all seniors' budgets at risk. Single seniors face even more pronounced challenges with more than half (55 percent) at risk with respect to their monthly housing expenses." In the Senior Economic Security Index the researchers developed, housing costs were one of five key measures, along with health care, household budget, home equity, and household assets. A shocking 78 percent of people sixty-five and over were economically vulnerable, according to this analysis.[3]

A federal report found 40 percent of households with older people (either older homeowners or older occupants) had housing difficulties. The most common problem was high cost, meaning more than 30 percent of household income was spent on housing. Worse, this problem was growing significantly. In addition, roughly one in twenty older people lived in physically inadequate housing, by US standards, lacking full plumbing or proper heating for example.[4]

A study by the Department of Housing and Urban Development found that 1.3 million renters over age sixty-two had "worst case" housing situations in 2009, meaning that either they were paying over half their income on rent and/or living in dilapidated housing.[5]

As a way to ease living expenses, homesharing has gone on casually in many cities since World War II. Still, American devotion to single-family housing has long made shared housing somewhat suspect—okay for college kids, perhaps, but not what mature adults should do. The 1996 book *Under One Roof: Issues and Innovations in Shared Housing* argues against "our exclusive attachment to the single (nuclear) family dwelling and our corresponding neglect of shared housing arrangements for the numerous households that do not fit the prototype of the nuclear family." In addition to the type of homesharing described earlier in this chapter, some shared housing programs involve a large home managed by a public agency or nonprofit, where each person rents a room and shares common space. In this option, the book continued, "When residents voluntarily collaborate in the design, management, and use of shared accommodations, they can overcome the indignity of necessity in modest yet meaningful ways. Shared housing arrangements provide an important complement to conventional housing options."[6] According to NSHRC, there are thirteen "shared living residence" programs in seven states.

Affordable Living for the Aging (ALA), based in Los Angeles, operates several homes, each with nine to fourteen residents aged fifty-five and older. Each individual has his or her own bedroom and bath, with living room and kitchen used in common. The homes are in desirable neighborhoods and are rehabbed to blend into the surroundings rather than appear institutional. Many of the residents are still working, explains Rachel Caraviello, ALA vice president of programs and services, and they must have a low enough income to qualify for affordable housing. The rent is $495 to $590 a month—a bargain for the Los Angeles area. "[Residents] come and go, and support one another and get more and more comfortable with the community over time," Rachel said.

Because of the long waiting list for these homes and the high cost of renovation and construction, ALA has also embraced homesharing through a matchmaking service. Rachel admits that it's a labor-intensive process. ALA matches just fifty home providers with home seekers a year; "a shamefully small amount," she said.

To expand opportunities, ALA sponsored a national symposium in 2012 for homesharing programs to learn from each other. Part of the challenge is to normalize homesharing as a legitimate option for people to consider. One idea, said Rachel, is to mount a public relations campaign that focuses on the positive aspects: changing from "what am I giving up" by sharing a home to "what am I gaining," for example, sharing utility bills, DVD or music collections, or recipes.

"The outcome of the symposium was to emphasize that even though we're based in L.A., we have this bigger vision that what's good for the shared housing field is good for us," she said. "We think the time is right to push hard at it and build capacity up at the national level and let people know it's our commitment." They also hope to convince funders to invest in field initiatives "and help us grow up. Not to shed our grassroots image, but to be more coordinated in a way that's better for all of us."

Although housesharing is something homeowners can do on their own through online services such as Craig's List, programs operated by nonprofit agencies like ALA offer security to potential home providers. Program staff and volunteers conduct background checks on homeseekers, interview people to help find the right match, and provide an avenue for mediation if problems arise.

One such program is run by St. Ambrose in Baltimore, which has been helping low- and moderate-income families struggling to buy homes or avoid foreclosure for fifty years. In the 1980s, St. Ambrose created a program to facilitate homesharing. "One of the employees had this idea to start homesharing to give the elderly homeowner the ability to age in place and preserve the housing stock in Baltimore," explained counselor Annette Leahy Maggitti. "With one elderly person in the home, things start to get run down. Sometimes people are lonely, and depression sets in. Or they need more income to keep the house up."

For "Sue," a widow, renting rooms to people who have been screened by St. Ambrose has given her enough extra income to make improvements to her home, such as making it more energy efficient. She's had nineteen people rent rooms over the years, with the longest staying five years. One of her favorites was a physician from Beijing, who had come to do research at Johns Hopkins. "He was a breath of fresh air," said Sue. "He was so helpful and talented in his own right. He was savvy in a lot of handyman kinds of things. A couple of the people have been that way."

Getting help with small household chores is one benefit of shared housing. But so too is the chance to meet new people. "To find and be enriched by their cultures, it has been very enriching in my own life," Sue said.

Not everyone has worked out, she added. "You have to be aware that people come from all kinds of backgrounds. You don't know a person until you live with them. So you get some surprises. If you're willing to take a chance it could work out."

According to a survey of homesharing programs by NSHRC, more than one-third of homeshares involve bartering of services in exchange for greatly reduced rent. Typically, the home provider is older and often needs help with chores such as lawn mowing, snow shoveling, or doing light housework. They may need transportation or help with errands and shopping. In some cases, the agreement is for a certain number of hours of help a week. The bartering component can be invaluable to the low-income home seeker but challenging to manage as well.

Openness and flexibility are key to successful homesharing, "It's difficult because it's not a relationship we naturally understand," said HomeShare Vermont's Kirby Dunn. "Usually you live with family. To live with an unrelated person is a pretty unique experience, and then add in some expectation of barter, which is kind of undefined. When are you hanging out having dinner versus when are you on the clock?" The older person may assume they're just in friendly companionship, while the younger may assume he's fulfilling his work expectation. "It's a hard balance to find. When people do start looking at the hours and counting the hours, it's not going to work—there has to be the fluidity a little bit. It takes a certain amount of flexibility and not everyone is flexible, because it's change. For both parties, it's probably not their first choice—nobody's jumping up and down saying 'I wish I could have someone living in the spare bedroom.' And on the other side, they're thinking, 'I'd rather have my own place.'"

Vermont has two sister nonprofit programs that offer homesharing services. HomeShare Vermont (originally called Project Home) in the northwest Burlington region was founded in 1982, followed by Home Share Now in central Vermont in 2003.

"We do outcome surveys, and we find over 50 percent of people say they are happier, they're sleeping better, they're calling their families less often for help, they're getting out more," said Kirby. "If I could give you a drug and say you'll be sleeping better, and feel healthier and happier, you'd pay anything for that. We're social beings—we're really not meant to live alone."

At the same time, HomeShare Vermont has found that many people are resistant to trying homesharing. "You think 'I'm giving up my independence, my privacy, I'm losing control, and I'm losing the familiar' which as we get older gets harder and harder to do," Kirby said. "Change is happening all around us, and we want it to stop. But for the people who make a go of it, and get over that first couple months and build that bond, then it's like magic."

Unfortunately, said Amy Noyes, communications director of Home Share Now, there is often a stigma associated with housesharing. Some think home providers are "infirm." "Our biggest challenge is, a lot of people have an [incorrect] idea of what homesharing is. We're trying to break those molds to show them it doesn't have to look a particular way. Another challenge is, people think 'wow that's such a great idea,' but they don't think it's a great idea for *themselves*—but for society, their community. They can think of people who would really benefit from it—they don't think, 'hey that could be me.'"

In 2012, HomeShare Vermont was able to keep sixty-five older adults in their own homes and out of nursing homes. Home Share Now has also helped keep people independent. The program began after an older man approached the Montpelier Housing Task Force with the idea of housesharing. Much of their area is rural and escaped some of the peaks and valleys of the recession and housing crisis. But they have been hit with high home heating prices, which can push homeowners to seek renters to help pay the energy bills. The organization's goal: create affordable housing options with positive impacts on the community and the environment.

According to Amy, in 2011 Home Share Now matched ninety individuals "in safe, secure homeshares." She continued, "Eighty-four percent of our participants were low income, an increase from years prior, and approximately 22 percent receive Medicaid." Nearly one third were sixty-five or older. "Homesharing enables an increase in eating home cooked meals, a greater capacity to save for retirement or pay off college debt, a way for young people to succeed in a financial climate where entry-level wages are not enough to meet financial demands, an increase in social interactions, and a reduction in energy expenses due to shared utilities and transportation."

In 2011 Home Share Now kept eleven people out of a nursing home, for an estimated savings of more than half a million dollars annually, Noyes said. For example, one couple who were active community volunteers became homebound after losing their ability to drive. They called Home Share Now, hoping to find someone who could live with them in exchange for transportation. Before the homeshare match could be completed, though, the woman fell and broke her leg and ended up in a nursing home to recuperate. The nursing home would not discharge her unless there was someone in the home besides her husband, who was in his nineties. Home Share Now immediately got to work finding the couple a good match, and the woman was able to return home.

"Traditionally the home providers have been older," Amy said. "Often with older people who are alone, it's to have a protective presence there, if they fall down in the night."

Often, home providers are not looking for a companion, but they find that friendship evolves. "They say, 'I don't want a best friend, I'm just looking to rent my extra room. I don't want to have meals with them. They can come and go as they please,'" Amy said. "Then they find they really like each other and like spending time with each other. We had a homeshare match move to Connecticut together. The older woman sold her home and was moving to Connecticut where some adult children lived, and she said, 'I can't leave you, I like you so much.' Her homeshare match said, 'I'll come with you.' The whole family loves her."

Kirby of HomeShare Vermont herself is a homesharer and wouldn't have it any other way. She began during a time when she was recently divorced. Her mother was ill, living in another location, and Kirby was helping care for her as well as working full-time, managing her own home, and taking care of her pets. She decided to share her house in order to get some help. "It's been great," she said. "Every once in a while things can go kerflooey—I've cried when one person moved out, and I was happy when others moved out. It's a mix, but I keep doing it. I think it's good for me, and it's nice to have the light on when you come home some nights and not worry about the house when you go on vacation. I do think it's a great thing."

CHAPTER 11

The New Family
Balancing Togetherness and Privacy

Since prehistoric times, humans have banded together in family groups, helping each other through the stages of life. New anthropological research suggests that beginning some thirty thousand years ago, as humanity began to live past thirty years old, the role of grandparents became critical to a family's health and well-being. Elders' wisdom and experience enabled them to teach younger generations how to locate scarce water, forage for food or identify poisonous plants, and pass on tool-making and artistic skills.[1]

For tens of millennia and continuing today in much of the world, extended families live together as the norm. Yet in the United States that all changed, as working people migrated for jobs, family farms went under, or students went off to college and never returned to the fold. Even those who did not leave their hometowns began setting up their own households when they became adults, rather than remaining with their parents and siblings. When baby boomers came of age, multigenerational families living together reached their nadir. The percentage of multigenerational family households plunged from 24.7 in 1940 to 12.1 in 1980. In the United States between 1940 and 2008, 1970 had the fewest people—twenty-six million—living in multigenerational households.[2]

In recent times, though, there's been a shift in the other direction. In 2010 the portion of multigenerational households rose to 16.1 percent. By 2011, more than fifty-one million Americans—one in six—lived in multigenerational households, a 10 percent increase since the recession began in 2007.[3] (It should be noted that researchers define multigenerational households differently—some count those with three or more generations living together, while others count those with two generations of related adults.)

The living situation of older people has been a rollercoaster since the early twentieth century—going from 57 percent living with their extended families in 1900, to 17 percent in the 1980s and 1990s, and now edging up to 20 percent.[4] As the aging population swells, researchers project this trend will continue.

According to a 2010 Pew report, *The Return of the Multigenerational*

Family Household, family members are increasingly moving in together for a variety of reasons, from mortgage foreclosures, to unemployment of young adults, to looking out for elders. Immigrant and African American families have a strong tradition of living in multigenerational households. Nationally, roughly one-quarter of Latinos (22 percent), African Americans (23 percent) and Asians (25 percent) live in multigenerational households, compared to 13 percent of whites.[5]

Although living with extended kin has ancient roots, modern families are changing how they live together. When they can afford a large enough dwelling, today's multigenerational households are more intentional about maintaining boundaries and honoring privacy. They often seek reciprocal relationships, where each has a valued role to play.

Three Units/Four Generations

A poster family for intergenerational living is the Cardozo clan in San Francisco. I met Laurie, of my generation, at the Morning Due coffee shop in the Castro district. It was a bustling café serving Fair Trade organic coffee, with artisan pottery and oil paintings on the walls. After ordering croissants and mugs of coffee, we settled in for conversation. Laurie, a tall, attractive woman with curly brown hair beginning to gray, was full of humor and confidence.

She grew up in Minneapolis and never expected that her extended family would eventually all live under one roof, once she and her siblings were grown. Unlike the familiar pattern of the young adults pulling up roots, her parents were the ones to move, leaving the Twin Cities for San Francisco in 1975 where her father worked in the book-selling trade. Her parents bought a large house that had previously been converted into two full apartments and an in-law suite, thinking that the rental income would help out.

In 1981, when Laurie and her husband decided to move West to work for the family business, her father suggested they rent the apartment above. "My mom said no—that's how she grew up, in an intense and large Jewish family that she ran away from," Laurie recalled. But she and her husband and children did move in, and "Thirty-one years later, I haven't left."

Today, the house is comprised of Laurie and her husband on the top floor, her parents in the middle, and her daughter, son-in-law, and their baby in the in-law suite on the lower level, making it four generations. "I hope this arrangement will continue on into the future, for many generations," said Laurie.

To her, the privacy and boundaries that come with each having their own unit makes it all work. "I couldn't do it otherwise," she said. On Friday nights they all gather to have dinner, but otherwise they do not share meals.

Like every group of people I interviewed, the family hits rough patches now and then. Laurie recalled the time when her father was in his early sixties and went to Findhorn, a spiritual community in Scotland. He returned insistent that he had found "the spiritual answers to life," and that the entire family should follow suit. After a few sessions of family therapy, they were able to move on. "We all have our quirks," she said. "We process it, and leave my parents alone. In true Midwestern fashion, no one likes to confront each other."

She acknowledged how fortunate her family is. For one, her daughter is a social worker who is used to dealing with difficult issues when they arise. Moreover Laurie's son-in-law is a home health aide who not only has a flexible schedule but is entirely comfortable and skilled in dealing with the age-related problems of her parents, who are now in their eighties. He and Laurie's husband, now retired, provide much of the childcare, while she and her daughter work outside the home as a high school teacher and social worker, respectively.

"My son-in-law takes the baby up to see my parents daily," she said. "And I've gotten to watch my daughter be a new mom. When I was a new mom, I was alone in a city in Minnesota." The nuclear family living alone, she concluded, makes no sense and reflects poorly on the US culture of individualism. In contrast, she said, "In our counter-culture stuff a lot of us are trying to stay more connected to our children and our parents. The sense of community is really important."

That she views this deep sense of family connection as counter-cultural is somewhat ironic, since so often baby boomers were labeled the "me generation," portrayed as a bunch of selfish ingrates thumbing their nose at authority in adolescence and now acting as "greedy geezers" defending their Social Security and Medicare.

Laurie's own grandparents all wound up in nursing homes. The places weren't "horrific," she said, "but if we can take care of [our elders], I think we should."

That view represents the majority opinion, according to a 2012 survey of how different generations (baby boomers and younger) view family responsibility. Among baby boomers, 55 percent thought adult children had a strong or absolute responsibility to ask their parents to live with them if they needed caregiving help, with another 26 percent believing this was a moderate responsibility. They were somewhat less charitable about taking their parents in if they were having financial difficulty—47 percent thought it was a strong responsibility and 28 percent thought moderate.[6]

It would be a mistake, though, to view intergenerational living, as a one-way "take care of the old folks" street. Modern grandparents, among them a growing number of baby boomers, are exceedingly generous to their grandchildren, according to a 2012 MetLife Mature Market Institute study. Some 62 percent helped out their grandchildren financially, for clothing and education for example. The average gift was more than $8,000 total for their grandchildren, and more than half the grandparents gave more than $5,000.[7]

The study also found that many grandparents were generous with their time and attention. Nearly one-third of grandparents babysat for their grandchildren five days a week, and one in ten provide full-time care for a grandchild. Twenty percent lived in multigenerational households.[8] Happily, the most frequently cited reason why people took care of their grandchildren was that they enjoyed doing so, followed by "so their parents can work."

The traditional role of grandparents as wise counselors, givers of unconditional love, and transmitters of strong values can be strengthened when families live together or in close proximity. In the MetLife study, a majority of grandparents saw themselves as the ones to pass on such values as honesty, good behavior, self-sufficiency, higher education, and good health habits. Twenty-two percent said they provided care to their grandchildren *in order* to pass on family values.

In Laurie's family, her parents have always been close to their grandchildren, as a result of living under one roof. Laurie remembers her daughter as a picky eater who, if Laurie's dinner didn't sound appetizing, would run upstairs to grandma and grandpa's to check out their menu, and if she gave that a thumbs down she knew her aunt in the basement apartment would make her what she wanted.

"For me, as a mother and now as a grandmother, it's so much easier and so much better for the kids to have more loving adults around them," Laurie said. "When my daughter was frightened by my son's health [her son had a seizure disorder], she'd run and climb in my parents' bed. That's the best thing—seeing what it does for children. As a high school teacher I see that the youth want adults to care for them and help them. My kids would do crazy things as teenagers. They would know there would always be at least one adult who would be there for them."

The In-Law Suite

Families choose to live together in all sorts of configurations and for all sorts of reasons. Unlike Laurie's family, whose younger members moved into the elders' home, in many cases the elder moves into the adult child's home. That was the case for Cheri and her wife, Ann, who live in a large house outside Grove City, Ohio, with an in-law suite for Cheri's eighty-four-year-old mother, Della. "I live alone, but they're there if something would happen to me," said Della. "It works out really well for us."

Della grew up in a large farm family in South Dakota, with seven sisters and four brothers and attended a one-room school. She never dreamed she would live to old age. Most of her family died in their early seventies, and she had always assumed she would too.

She first moved to Columbus and rented a house with another woman, but there were problems. "Cheri thought it would be best to get out of that situation," she said. She had worked as a registered nurse all her life, but her retirement prospects were dim. Divorced and with substance abuse problems, she had very little money to live on. Cheri and Ann offered to share their home with her. Twenty years and two homes later, the two generations still lived together. Della contributed $8,000 to the down-payment on their first house, and later helped out with utilities.

As an extended family, they knew from the beginning they wanted to set clear boundaries. Early on, Della often cooked dinner for Cheri and Ann, who were free to take their plates to their own part of the house if they wished. As Della grew older, cooking became more of a challenge, but she still helped out as best she could. She took care of Cheri and Ann's cat and dog, for example, when the couple went out of town.

Their friends often included Della in dinner invitations, and a few would come by to visit her. Della, who had no friends left of her own, was grateful for the companionship of family. "There was a little church close by, and I met several ladies there and was in a craft club," she said. "At that time, these ladies were all older. They died one by one." She also used to meet former nursing colleagues once a month for lunch, but physical ailments—her own and her friends'—made it impossible to keep up.

"I like having my own space," she said of the separate apartment. "I really feel like this is my place." She decorated however she wished, and had her own deck to be outside. I asked her if Ann and Cheri would approve of her having a "gentleman friend." "That would be nice!" she laughed. "I'm sure they would let me know if they approved."

I later spoke individually to Cheri and Ann. Ann recalled that when Cheri first proposed the idea of her mother moving in with them, Ann had no problem with it. "I was clear about specific boundaries," she said. "I knew this was not a trial—this was going to be it."

She knew that Della's living situation was not good and neither were her finances. So Ann appreciated that Della helped with their first down payment. "We all benefited, and it's still working," she said. In the beginning, Della was in her sixties and still "vital," said Ann. "She cooked for us, she did our laundry."

But the house design was not ideal. Della had a humble basement bedroom and bath. When Cheri found their current home with an in-law suite, they decide to move, even though it meant a longer commute.

"It's important from a family perspective," Ann said. "We get to see extended family more than we would normally. Having Della with us draws the family together."

When I asked what would happen if Della needed more care, Ann responded, "We're winging it."

One issue that caused friction was Della's smoking. Ann and Cheri insisted that she smoke by her sink or on the deck. "We caught her a couple times," Ann said. "We had very strong words. My concern is fire. This is our life, and she's part of the household."

Still, Ann added, "Della's a peach. I don't know if you'd get that every time. My grandmother lived with my family when I was a child. My mom and grandmother didn't get along all the time—she was my dad's mom."

She and Cheri tried to encourage Della to get out and meet friends and offered to take her to the senior center. But, they concluded, "She's a homebody. She wouldn't ever go," Ann said.

For Cheri, the idea of housesharing came after several occasions when they had to help her mother with problems stemming from her alcoholism and addiction. "I thought maybe it made sense to think ahead," she said.

Cheri felt good about their current living situation. Her mother "loves the birds. She has a big bedroom, a nice bathroom, a kitchen/dining room, and a nice big living room, with her own fireplace. On her deck the grandkids help her with flowers, and she waters the plants and fills the birdfeeders."

Della also got a lot of pleasure from Toby, a deaf cat whom she adopted after finding the teeny white ball of fur up in a tree. The cat, said Cheri, had gone from needing Della's care to being Della's caretaker, giving her companionship and plenty of lap time.

As Della grew somewhat frailer, they began to cook for her. During the week, she ate in her apartment, and on the weekends they dined together.

Cheri's niece and nephew chose to go to college nearby to be closer to Della, who enjoys cooking for her grandchildren. "My mom's life in the last few years is better than ever," Cheri said. Her mother has always been open to

Cheri being a lesbian, and was happy when she and Ann got married. "Ann has helped support her," Cheri said. "They have a great relationship." Ann helped Della through recovery from substance abuse.

"In twenty years, there's never been a period of time that we thought this isn't working," Cheri said. "Still today, she watches the dog for us. She lets repair people in. And we're emotional support for her. If she lived somewhere else, it would be much harder to deal with if she needed help. It's been beneficial for me—my mother is my friend too."

The main advice she and Ann give to families considering living together is to talk about rules and boundaries. Early on, for example, Della would go through their mail or open their packages. They were able to work through that.

At the end of our conversation, I had the chance to talk to Liz, Della's granddaughter. "My mom [Cheri's sister] appreciated this when Cheri and Ann opened their doors to my grandmother," she said. "We don't have to worry or think about putting her in assisted living."

Liz laughed that there may come a day when she would be helping out her own parents, Della, and Cheri and Ann. "The running joke is I'll get all of them," she said. "I'll have a commune or a farm. This has been really nice for me. Before I only saw Grandma once a year, when I was in Montana. When I come to visit, I'm not pressured to see all of them. We try to take Grandma out on her own. She still makes the best cookies in the world. All the grandkids come and help her with Christmas cookies."

Recently, I checked in with Cheri to find out how Della was doing. She had died a few months earlier, from an aneurysm. "She lived with us until the day she died," Cheri wrote, "and frankly I still miss her every day."

The GRAMS

As Cheri and Ann described, having boundaries and discussing them up front is important for families making the decision to live in the same household.

Social psychologist Susan Newman, author of *Under One Roof Again: All Grown Up and (Re)learning to Live Together Happily*, agrees. "There are a lot of questions they should ask as they're thinking about moving in together," she said in an interview, assuming there is a choice and that the move is not prompted by truly dire circumstances. "What they should ask themselves first is why are we doing this? How am I going to feel about this move? Am I going to feel I'm at the mercy of my children? How can we make this equitable?"

If the older person or couple is moving in with their adult children, she said, they should make a financial contribution as Della did, such as helping pay to fix up an in-law suite. "The older generation wants to contribute," she said. "Even if you don't really need their money, take it anyway. It makes them feel they are part of the building process, and they have some ownership in this move."

That was the case for another family. Anne, at sixty-five, pulled up stakes in San Diego and moved north to the Bay Area to be near her two children. She had been in San Diego for thirty years and had a successful psychotherapy practice.

"One day my son called and said, 'Mom you always wanted to live in the Bay Area.' They were getting ready to have their first baby," she explained. "He said, 'We need you here, and you don't want to miss your first grandchild.'"

With that, she decided to move, gradually scaling back her therapy practice as she slowly made the transition. She invited me over to the lovely house she purchased with her son and daughter-in-law. Together they had planned an addition that included a family room on the main floor and a small apartment below for Anne, a hip-looking grandmother wearing blue jeans, who was heading out to canvass for President Obama's reelection after our interview.

"I had a lot of trepidation, as you can imagine," she said of the move. "I had never lived in one room before. I had piles and piles of junk from not only my life, but my mother's and grandmother's. I didn't know what it would be like to live so near my kids and grandkids."

She knew that she wanted a separate entrance to her space, but was conflicted over whether to have her own kitchen. She's glad now that she doesn't. She goes out a lot, and when she's at home she enjoys eating with the family. "My daughter-in-law and I love and respect each other, luckily," she said. "She wants to be in charge of cooking, and I don't like to cook. I do the dishes, and she doesn't mind that." That gives her daughter-in-law and son the opportunity to be with the children after supper.

"One thing that's awkward is that if I want to have people for dinner, I wait until they're gone for the weekend," she said.

Initially, she did a lot of childcare. Her grandchildren, ages three and five, are now in school until three o'clock each afternoon, then she takes care of them for two hours during the week and some on the weekends. During the day, Anne found she had too much time on her hands, so she volunteered on the political campaign and joined the Berkeley Community Chorus, which is open to all ages and abilities. At the time of our conversation, the chorus was preparing to tour in Europe and take a master class with the head of the Vienna Boys' Choir.

She showed me her space, a snug apartment with a desk, bed, and bathroom. The apartment opens on to the backyard full of fruit trees and tomato plants.

"I've made a few compromises," she said. She had longed to live in Berkeley, her alma mater, and be able to walk to the campus, but the other two wanted to live in Oakland, which was more affordable and had lots of young families. She also acknowledged that every bump in the road makes her heart clutch—"When there's tension in the house, I can't just go home," she laughs.

But, she said, the arrangement works beautifully and she hopes to stay there indefinitely. The neighbors include her as part of the family at get-togethers. I ask if she's thought about what would happen if she grew frail or unable to care for herself. "We didn't really discuss this in depth," she said. "If it turns out it would be better for me to be someplace else, I'll move. My son has said, 'If you're sick I'd much rather take care of you here than drive across town.'"

The bottom line, she said, is, "We like each other. That makes a big difference. And I don't need to be in charge."

Anne is part of a close-knit group of women who chose to move in order to live near their children and grandchildren in the greater San Francisco area. They've dubbed themselves the GRAMS, for Grandmothers Relocating After Midlife Successfully.

At a gathering they'd organized on my behalf, they shared their stories about what this huge transition has meant in their lives. Each had taken a somewhat different path.

My friend Karen, an artist, and her husband had moved from my hometown and bought a parcel of land outside Santa Cruz together with their son and daughter-in-law. The latter moved into a modest home on the property, and Karen and Frank built a small, energy-efficient home just steps away. Their other son and daughter-in-law live a few miles away. Each son has one little boy.

Mary Helen had retired from a scientific career with the pharmaceutical industry in Salt Lake City to become a weaver, moving to Berkeley where she lives in an apartment one mile from her daughter, son-in-law, and grandchildren.

Judith moved from Seattle in order to be near her two daughters, their husbands, and her six grandchildren, aged nine months to eighteen years. She lives on the first floor of a beautiful old house on a corner lot in Berkeley, where we were meeting.

Mary, a long-time public school administrator, and her husband also moved from Maryland and now live next door to their daughter.

Sitting on comfortable chairs in Judith's living room, the women shared heart-felt thoughts on their new lives. The group formed after initially meeting each other at a neighborhood park as they were taking care of their grandchildren. As they chatted at the park, they realized how much they had in common and eventually formed the GRAMS. They had been meeting monthly for four years.

"The GRAMS have been lifesavers for my sanity," said Mary. Her daughter had urged them to move, saying she'd like to be a support for them as they grew old. "So I took it that's what we're going to do. My husband came here reluctantly, and he remembers our conversations differently." While Mary loves being so close to their daughter, her husband has strict boundaries. He did not grow up in a close family, and it doesn't come naturally to him, she said. It was a difficult family transition, and for a time Mary suffered from depression. But they have gotten through it.

Mary Helen and Judith also had been urged by their children to move to the area. Five years earlier, Mary Helen's daughter said, "'We are going to have children, and I always pictured you in the picture,'" Mary Helen recalls. "We left it very open. But something inside me shifted then. I didn't know this was what I wanted until it was offered. I retired early and moved out here."

Judith's son-in-law told her, "You'll move down." At first she rented an apartment and came for frequent visits while still working in Seattle. After a time, she came for good. She has an especially close relationship with her oldest grandson, who has learning disabilities. He has always been her pal, and she helps tutor him. Both daughters live within a mile or so of her. Judith sees the younger one a couple of times a week, for childcare and dinner; the older she sees five times a week. "I'm very integrated with their lives," she said. Despite their close relationship, she has no desire to live with either of her daughters. But she has thought about getting a housemate.

Karen does a considerable amount of childcare for both her grandsons. One daughter-in-law has a demanding career as a chef and owner of three businesses. Karen's husband also helps with the kids and is a master gardener who tends the vegetables and fruit trees on the property. Karen feels they play a central and important role of support and stability in the family. But it has also been wrenching, as they left a strong network of close friends and other family members back East.

I asked the GRAMS about the challenges of moving to a new place at this time of life. "When you uproot your life you leave behind a lot of who you were as a person—the support, the friends," said Mary Helen.

"Your identity," Karen added.

"A lot of people aren't willing to do that," Mary Helen said. "It's uncomfortable to be a newcomer. You have to be prepared for that and realize half your neighbors may have their own dance cards full. You have to be confident or relentless enough to say, 'I'm going to make a place here.'"

"Is it worth it or not?" Karen said. "You did it, and there's no going back. The gifts are—I will die with no regrets. If I hadn't done it, I would have had regrets. I have found meaning in my new life. That's worth it."

I asked them if the grandchildren were the magnet, or if they would have moved anyway to be near their adult children. While the grandchildren were the immediate draw, they felt that being near their adult children was also compelling.

"I think it's essential to life," said Judith. "I have no regrets."

"I feel like I'm more alive now," said Karen. "I'd known for years I wanted to be near my kids, but fear held me back. Being near my kids is the center of my life. I believe this is about my spiritual development. We must say yes. And this whole move was what my body and soul wanted."

☙❧

Not everyone articulates such lofty reasons for moving in with family. Often it's something as mundane as needing to share the electric bill and rent or offering shelter when a family member suddenly loses his spouse or job or has a medical crisis. Or it simply feels like the way life should be.

The Murphy family, who recently moved to Maryland from Washington, DC, has always had one or more of their adult children living with them. They moved to a roomy house with a basement apartment a block from their two daughters' small business, a bakery and café.

"The café took over all of our lives," said Caitlin, the baker and co-owner of the business. Because of a vision problem, Caitlin is unable to drive, so her parents' new home allows her to walk to work and for them to pitch in at the café on the spur of the moment.

Caitlin's mother, Sharon, said her husband had grown up in the model of the 1950s, with a nuclear family and grandparents who moved to nursing homes when they grew old. She, on the other hand, grew up "dirt poor" in Detroit. For her, "It's a way of being, that grandparents live with you," she said, "or adult kids who lost their job or their partner."

She recalls her own grandmother who in her eighties was still working in the family pub. She would rise at four a.m. and walk through East Detroit in order to make the meat pies. "It was endearing," she said. "It didn't matter if she were slow or even if someone else could make the meat pies better. She was part of the family and people appreciated her."

Sharon and her husband founded a nonprofit to provide transitional housing for families in crisis, especially for new immigrants and refugees. They raised their children in a large house where some of the families lived, so life was always full of people and hubbub.

Sharon grows impatient with our generation who she believes spends too much time "processing" ad nauseam such decisions as allowing your adult children to move home for a while. "I think it's the greatest gig in the world to have kids and to have them want to live with you when they're adults," she said. "Our generation feels they need to understand everything. It's so much more fun not to invest energy in that."

As she's building up her business, Caitlin said she could not afford to live on her own. "I put on fifteen pounds when I went home," she laughed. "My mom cooks every night. My dad replaces my light bulbs. It's great." But she admits that at first she struggled with being thirty years old and moving back home.

"It's a legitimate question, but then you have to let it go," her mother said. "That's more about [other people's] perceptions."

Caitlin is realizing that more and more of her friends and customers are making a similar choice. "I enjoy the fact that I can hang out with my parents when they're strong and healthy," she said. "We hang out every day I'm off. We're best friends."

Sharon nods, but she said she knows she has to keep clear about when she needs to separate emotionally from her "mom" role. When she gave Caitlin a ride for a medical consultation, for example, Sharon had to leave the doctor's office to keep from putting in her two cents. "She would have decked me if I'd spoken out," she said, as Caitlin nodded.

They both stress that living together is not a bed of roses. They bicker and fight and drive each other crazy. Then they let it go. Sharon recalls one of the arguments that Caitlin and her sister had over their shared business. "It was horrible," she said. "I was worried it would ruin our family. I was driving to work praying to God, praying to the grandmothers. I was a wreck. Then I come back home at the end of the day and they're laughing and everything's fine."

PART III

Getting from Here to There

Despite our best efforts and intentions, age happens. For some of us, growing old will be more sweet than bitter. Our gait may slow, words might escape us from time to time, our hearing or vision may be less sharp. But in the important ways, life continues to have pleasure and meaning. We'll stay closely connected with our loved ones, feel valued, appreciate the world around us, and find meaning day to day. We may not be wealthy, but we don't worry that we'll go hungry or lose our home. We can thank some combination of living sensibly, inheriting the right genes, and dumb luck, if we are able to live long and die comfortably in our favorite chair.

But then there are the rest of us. We may—or may not—have lived pretty much like our fortunate neighbor or relative, but the cards we were dealt turned up a different hand altogether. Our memories gradually elude us, becoming so deeply buried we can no longer access them, until finally even remembering to lift our fork is beyond us. Our heart or lungs may fill with fluid, or we may find ourselves inexplicably falling. We may have a stroke or Parkinson's disease that leaves us so debilitated we simply cannot manage to live at home, certainly not without assistance. Few of us have the financial resources to pay for full-time in-home care, and families may not be able to help out as much as we need. And so we end up in the places that we most dread.

Although it's far more soothing to expect the first scenario, we are wise to contemplate the latter. I have yet to meet a single soul whose goal is to end up in a nursing home. So what is our Plan B?

Are our homes and neighborhoods suitable for our aging selves? Do we know how we will pay for help if we need it and where that help will come from? Are we open to new technology being installed in our homes, some of which might seem intrusive? These are the questions we need to be thinking about, well before the need arises.

CHAPTER 12

Design for Life

Building Homes and
Neighborhoods That Serve Us

Remodeler Stephen Hage is a man with a mission.

It began twenty years ago, when he was having a beer after work with a friend. Steve was at a crossroads. He and his business partner had parted company, and Steve felt dissatisfied with his remodeling work. "I thought, do I want to keep doing granite countertops?" he recalls. "I could. But do I want to?" His friend told him he should look up a guy named Louis Tenenbaum, an expert in the emerging field of aging in place.

One thing led to another and Steve ended up working with Tenenbaum for a decade. "It became my life's work," he said. "It was what I was supposed to do. It combined my building skills with my sense of ministry—of wanting to reach people."

Most people probably don't imagine such fervor coming from the guy who installs their grab bars. But to Steve, the idea of making your home environment serve your needs is an important and meaningful goal that he can help you achieve.

In the beginning, he said, "We were a voice in the desert." He did all he could think of to market the idea of adapting people's homes. He contacted discharge planners of hospitals and rehabilitation centers to no avail. "The real problem has been a disconnect between the medical and the practical," he said. Hospitals blithely discharge patients to their homes which can be accidents waiting to happen. Individuals are left to their own devices to decide how to make their homes safe—or not. Too often, the result is people fall, sending them back to the hospital. In fact, one in three people over sixty-five fall each year, according to the National Council on Aging.[1] That can lead to a cascade of events that end in the nursing home or in death.

To help prevent such problems, Steve Hage started his small company, Strategies for Independent Living. I met with him in his home office, a few blocks from mine, along with my friend Isabelle Schoenfeld, a federal government retiree who also wants to spread the gospel of aging in place and universal design. We began by talking about the language of design—and how the ongoing denial of aging can be a barrier to change.

"The term 'aging in place' itself is a problem," Steve said. "Anyone over sixty will resist that language." Still, he does see change, and a new vocabulary emerging. He and others are experimenting with different terms to describe what they do: "Smart design," "livability," "visitability," "adaptability," and so on. A home with "visitability," explained Steve, basically means that someone in a wheelchair would be able to enter your house for a visit and use the bathroom while there.

I would have loved to have had "visitability" in our home when my mother was alive. After frequent falls and broken bones, she spent the last year of her life using a wheelchair and had to move to the assisted living building on the campus of her retirement community. To our frustration, it was very difficult for her to come visit us, even though we were just a half hour apart. Our home has eight steps to the front porch, and even though we have two bathrooms on the first floor, neither is accessible for someone in a wheelchair.

Hopefully, Mom's predicament will become a rarity over time. Increasingly, designers and architects are thinking in terms of universal design—planning homes that work for everyone. In Australia, the construction industry adopted voluntary standards to make all new housing accessible by 2020.[2] The standards, developed by the housing industry and disability advocates, set as a baseline that new homes will have a stepless entry, wide doors and halls, a ground-floor bathroom, a "hobless" shower without a rim on the floor to allow wheelchair access, and reinforced walls to allow grab bars to be installed.

Jon Sanford, director of the Center for Assistive Technology and Environmental Access at the Georgia Institute of Technology, explains the difference between universal design and accessibility. "Accessibility by definition is designed for people with disabilities," he said. "Universal design by definition is design for everybody, including people with disabilities. Accessible design is primarily about removing barriers in the environment, where with universal design there aren't any barriers to start with."

Universal design, as its name implies, is marketed to all homeowners as a comfortable and convenient home plan that doesn't call attention to itself. In contrast, accessibility modifications for aging in place are typically more noticeable.

Isabelle Schoenfeld said she explains to clients how universal design means a home is more comfortable and works better for everyone. For example, having kitchen counters of different heights means a child can work comfortably at a lower counter to do homework or an art project, and later, if needed, an adult in a wheelchair could use that space for food preparation. "Everybody in the household benefits," she said. "I think universal design should be promoted at all levels, from the initial building or remodeling, no matter your age or abilities. It makes good design sense."

In the United States, the trend toward universal design is growing, if not exactly snowballing. According to Bill Owens, a remodeler from the Columbus, Ohio, area who leads the National Association of Homebuilders' education program for Certified Aging in Place Specialists, "Every project we do, we go in with our universal-design glasses on."

Owens said he continues to be amazed at his customers' denial of aging. When his own mother was seventy-eight she told him she didn't need him to make such changes in her home, as such adaptations were for "old people." "You are not going to get very far if you go out and profess you're the best aging-in-place contractor," he said. "People don't want to buy your product—it's like selling caskets."

Nevertheless, he is seeing a lot of interest among contractors who want to receive NAHB's certification for aging in place. Other than green building, it is their most popular certification.

Owens believes, though, that we're far from a tipping point when it comes to universal design. "We're at the innovator stage," he said. While those who study trends say you need 25 percent market immersion before an idea really takes hold, he said, universal design has perhaps 5 percent of the market.

According to Owens, most requests for adaptations that remodelers receive involve the bathroom—removing bathtubs, which can be very difficult to get in and out of, and replacing them with low-threshold or no-threshold showers, and installing grab bars in the shower or around the toilet. Elevators, he added, are a tough sell to today's Depression-Era elders, who see a home elevator as "an absolute luxury." "They'd rather be forced out of their homes," he said.

Elevators range in price from $15,000 to $30,000, not counting building a shaft, which can easily bring the price to $50,000, depending on the home. Far more affordable are chair lifts, which can be installed for as little as $2,500 although customized ones for long or curving staircases can cost far more. Another option is a "Telecab," which doesn't need a shaft like an elevator but is more of a box that moves up and down, costing $16,000 to $20,000, according to Steve Hage.

Unlike universal design, Owens said aging-in-place adaptations are more familiar and more readily requested. "The problem with this is, nobody is interested in buying until they absolutely need it," he said. "It's too narrow of a market place. Universal design is a more proactive approach. We're not asking people to perform to their homes. We're trying to make the home perform better for the inhabitants. If we're more proactive and hit a larger share of the marketplace with some of these inclusions, you'd have more business than [relying on] someone who has an accident or illness or progressive condition."

Because of people's denial, contractors have to use some delicacy in approaching customers. "To begin an aging-in-place discussion, we'll build trust by saying, 'we understand the house comes up short,'" Owens said, rather than pointing out the client's own physical vulnerability.

To build consumer interest in universal design, NAHB is launching a new certification campaign, called Better Living Design. NAHB hopes consumers will someday equate the Better Living Design symbol with a more livable and comfortable home, much as they associate the EnergyStar icon with energy-efficient products. Despite these efforts, said Georgia Tech's Sanford, builders nationally are generally slow to change. "It's hard to get people on board," he said. "The biggest problem is that builders build the way they've always been building; everything is about cost. Even though they can spend extravagant amounts of money on one thing, they'll skimp on something else and say it's about cost." Customers, he adds, aren't much better. Often, simple changes could be made that would have minimal or no impact on cost. For example, to make a bathroom large enough to be used by someone in a wheelchair might require making a somewhat smaller bedroom, rather than adding to the total square footage of the home.

In addition to universal design and accessibility, NAHB has observed another new trend: an increase in multigenerational living. As discussed in Chapter 11, economic hard times during the recent recession and housing crisis, as well as an increase in immigrant families, have contributed to the growth in multigenerational homes. According to Stephen Melman, NAHB director of economic services, multigenerational living represents a "growing niche market, which is continuing to expand. We would anticipate the cultural [i.e., African American and immigrant families] demand would take a bigger share, even as the recession recedes."

He points to major builders, such as Pulte and Lennar, that are now building new homes with a separate small apartment that can be accessed from either the outside or a connecting inside door. Lennar calls its line of multigenerational housing "Next Gen." Some 600 square feet of a 3,000-square-foot home is for the "Next Gen Suite" that includes a living room, small kitchen with microwave/convection oven and space to eat, a bedroom, bath, and private patio. (Its ad shows three generations, holding hands in a circle and twirling gleefully around the grandparents' "home within a home" suite.) According to a 2012 *New York Times* article, Lennar already has one hundred communities in ten states with Next Gen homes, and it plans to include the model in all its developments.[3]

One potential stumbling block for those wanting to add apartments is overly-stringent zoning laws that favor single-family homes. Many localities, including Montgomery County where I live, claim to be supportive of aging in place, yet their housing codes have not kept up with changing needs, and getting licensed for an accessory apartment can be burdensome.

Even more difficult in terms of potential cost and zoning barriers are separate dwellings. One that has received considerable attention is the MEDCottage—a.k.a. "granny pod"—meant to house an elder who may need assisted living or nursing-home level care. The MEDCottage is a modular studio apartment that an adult child can plant in the backyard, fully equipped with sensors, a hospital bed, and other medical technology to keep an elder safe— but at a slight distance.

The cottage can be outfitted with all sorts of health-care and monitoring gizmos: a toilet that measures urine output; a "virtual companion" TV monitor that issues helpful "it's time to take your medication" reminders, as well as offering games and music; lighting at knee height to illuminate the floor at night to prevent falls; and a Hoyer lift to help move the person from bed to chair or toilet. Other companies are developing similar "senior sheds" as a *Wall Street Journal* article dubbed them.[4]

After a *Washington Post* story on MEDCottage, the company, N2Care, reportedly was swamped with inquiries.[5] At this writing, five have been sold. Of course even with all the tricked-out features, you still need caregivers. Ken Dupin of Blacksburg, Virginia, who created the product, has said his idea was to create a distinctly American way for families to participate in eldercare, one that offers privacy to the caregiver and the elder alike. Whether families will pay the $55,000–$125,000 cost (depending on which customized features you need) is unclear.

Other accessory dwelling units, as they're known, using universal design but without all the medical bells and whistles, are also becoming available. FabCab in Seattle has an eco-friendly 550-square-foot cabin made of Douglas fir with plenty of glass that includes a bathroom and kitchen as well as storage space. Larson Shores Architects in Oakland, California, has developed similar "Inspired In-Law" dwellings.

ℰℵℸ

An often overlooked piece of aging in place—and one that affects everyone in a house, less so in an apartment—is home maintenance. In a 2012 study, researchers at Georgia Tech interviewed forty-four older people to learn more about their home maintenance concerns.[6] Participants made 316 comments on challenges they encountered. The most common difficulties were in three categories: more than one-third were related to cleaning (e.g., vacuuming, changing the sheets, doing laundry, taking out the garbage), slightly less to outdoor work (mowing the lawn, cleaning the gutters, painting), and 16 percent were related to home upkeep (changing the furnace filter, replacing light bulbs, pest control, replacing the roof).

Some of these maintenance challenges were enough to push people to move to a retirement community or an apartment, even if their preference would be to remain in their own homes. The study concluded that maintenance could be addressed through a wide range of solutions, including improved home design, technology such as robotic cleaning machines, and products such as self-cleaning furnace filters. It also noted that elders should have a pool of paid and volunteer help to assist with home maintenance they can reach out to.

Home maintenance help is one of many practical reasons why aging in some sort of community makes so much sense. Examples of communities organizing volunteers to help with maintenance include many Villages, the Greenbelt Intergenerational Volunteer Exchange Service (GIVES) program, and Secure@Home's "Chore Corps" in Princeton. Some of these groups also vet contractors for heavier duty work such as roofing or HVAC repair, to ensure the older person gets a high quality, reasonably-priced job from a contractor. Other people who decide to share their home with family members, friends, or a tenant also work out arrangements so that the older person is relieved of many maintenance chores.

Communities That Work for Everyone

Even having the best-designed home, surrounded by a community of friends, is not the whole answer to aging in place. A growing and hopeful movement views neighborhoods and towns through the lens of meeting the needs of people of all ages. Though programs are called by various names—livable, life-long, age-friendly—their approaches are similar. The idea is to holistically look at what is needed for a good quality of life and to proactively design to meet those needs. This includes walkable neighborhoods with services and businesses that people want, transportation for those who don't drive, and an environment that is safe and clean. Creating a truly life-long community requires professionals from many disciplines—civic planning, health care, transportation, parks and recreation, and arts and culture—pooling their expertise.

Enormous challenges stand in the way. According to a major nationwide survey of communities, while many piecemeal programs had moved forward, few communities "had undertaken a comprehensive assessment to create a 'livable community' *for all ages*, including the diverse population of those age 65+" (italics theirs).[7]

The challenge is especially great in areas known for suburban sprawl. Those neighborhoods that were the dream of families from the 1960s on, with everyone having their own home and yard and typically two or more cars, can become deserts of isolation for elders.

Savvy advocates for older people soon realized that rather than lobbying for big, sometimes costly, changes that will benefit only one age group, it's much better to point out the advantages for everyone at all stages of life. The same curb cuts, accessible buildings, or wide store aisles that help an elder who uses a wheelchair are appreciated by young fathers pushing a stroller, a skier who has broken her leg, and a disabled young veteran. Nearby clinics, libraries, post offices, and shops appeal to everyone, as do parks with benches.

A number of top research centers are tackling the challenge of how to affordably adapt homes and neighborhoods to accommodate people as they grow more frail or have cognitive difficulties. At Penn State, Richard Behr was the founding director of the Smart Spaces Center, an interdisciplinary initiative aimed at helping baby boomers age in place, particularly those who are low to middle income. The Center viewed the challenge broadly, as a series of concentric circles beginning with an individual home then moving outward. "If you do something to just your house it might not be enough," Behr explained. "Your neighborhood has to accommodate aging in place as much as the house does. Perforating all these spaces is the information space—new technologies that could enhance information exchange. As you go further out, you could deal with public policy and health policy—societal space. And so we looked at this problem from a holistic standpoint."

The Smart Spaces Center partnered with the nonprofit Blueroof Technologies, in McKeesport, Pennsylvania, to create "Smart Cottages," simple homes that blended into an existing intergenerational neighborhood. Toward that end, Blueroof launched "McKIZ." The idea was to retrofit suitable homes or to build Smart Cottages, neighborhood by neighborhood, to allow intergenerational aging in place. "That's the way to do this," said Behr. "Don't segregate people into elder communities." Such neighborhoods would have a grocery and a "neighborhood nurses' station," where people could be seen for many of their medical needs.

"There are all kinds of things that can be done on a neighborhood scale," he said. "It's going to run contrary to a lot of trends like suburban sprawl and Walmart. Everything is becoming centralized—we need to decentralize it. Elders need to be able to walk to a grocery store, to walk to a community center that has a health care professional on call."

Philanthropists, public agencies, small nonprofits, and businesses are helping bring this vision to life throughout the country and indeed the world. The World Health Organization (WHO) created a program to foster "age-friendly cities," including New York and Portland, Oregon, to network and share resources and strategies. The program identifies eight key components on which communities might focus their efforts to become age-friendly:

- transportation
- housing
- social participation
- respect and inclusion
- civic participation and employment
- communication and information
- community support and health services
- outdoor spaces and buildings

There are dozens of ways that US communities are working to become age friendly. As the following examples illustrate, successful programs reach far beyond the usual senior service agencies to include a wide range of public interests. They are also committed to the long term.

Age-Friendly Business Certification

The nonprofit Elders in Action, based in Portland, Oregon, created a way to encourage businesses and agencies of all types to become more accessible and customer-friendly. Older volunteers evaluate the business for wheelchair and walker accessibility, lighting, large-print signs, and customer service. They call to make sure a real person answers the phone, one who speaks clearly and is able to give good directions, not only to drivers but to those traveling by public transportation. The grocery store New Seasons, for example, widened its aisles, lowered its plastic bag dispenser, made produce signs larger, and added comfy chairs for shoppers to rest. A large "age friendly" decal is on the store's front window, and the certification can be used in the company's advertising and promotion. In addition to the certification, Elders in Action offers training to businesses to improve service to customers of all ages, particularly those who are older. More than 325 businesses are certified as age-friendly, and many others have requested training. (The program originally was called "elder-friendly" but such is the prejudice against old people that Elders in Action changed the certification to "age-friendly," both to match the WHO designation, but also, executive director Leslie Foren said, because their marketing team found that businesses were not eager to have an "elder-friendly" decal on their door.)

From Sprawl to Walkability

Mableton, Georgia, has launched a demonstration project to test if elder-unfriendly sprawl can be transformed into a livable community.[8] The town has a forty-year plan that begins, interestingly, with a new elementary school. The idea is that if you make the town good for children and for elders it will be good for everyone. One big challenge is a very busy road that cuts through the town, carrying high-speed commuters passing through. To get from the library to the arts center just two hundred yards away requires a car, unless you want to risk a treacherous highway crossing on foot. The town's solution is to reconfigure the road, moving through-traffic to the center, bordered by green median strips with trees, and creating smaller outside lanes for local traffic. Rather than having to dash across the big road, pedestrians will only have to go short distances before reaching a safe spot. A new town square is also on the drawing board, and residents passed a new zoning code allowing for mixed-use development. As it designs more walkable spaces, Mableton is simultaneously creating buy-in from walking clubs. It used a process called Photovoice that invites residents to evaluate walking routes, using photographs and narrative to look at their community. Mableton also created a farmer's market and a large intergenerational community garden in the center of town.

"The reason Mableton is important is that it's the only example of a lifelong or livable community where they've taken a very broad-based approach—not just the physical, not just the social environment, not just the political environment, it's all of these things put together that make it a viable example of a livable community," said architect Jon Sanford, of Georgia Tech. And they're doing this in a town where "the physical environment was fighting against them from the start," he added.

Urban Transformation

Philadelphia, Pennsylvania, with one of the oldest populations among large cities, has developed an ambitious Age-Friendly Philadelphia (AFP) plan, based on the US Environmental Protection Agency's Aging Initiative model. Undergirding the plan are four key principles:

1. Social capital: Being active and connected in one's neighborhood
2. Flexible and accessible housing: Having the option to remain in one's home and/or community
3. Mobility: Having access to public transportation and a walkable environment
4. Healthy eating: Having fresh fruits, vegetables, and other nutritious foods available

This approach, which combines the built environment with social connections, confirms that the well-being of older adults is fostered by far more than their individual habits or access to medical care. "Consider an older adult who reports high social capital, whose home does not require major repairs, and who has access to transportation and to fresh fruits and vegetables. This older adult is far more likely to report being in excellent or good health; to experience few if any depressive symptoms in the week prior to being interviewed; to be more physically active; and to want to remain in his or her home for at least another ten years," according to a progress report on Philadelphia's efforts.[9]

AFP has met with over 150 organizations that do not traditionally work with older people, to raise awareness about how to better weave the lives of elders into the broader life of the community.

In the progress report AFP explains steps being taken by a wide range of agencies and nonprofits to bring each principle to life. For example, a survey found that while Philadelphia enjoys a ten-thousand–acre park system, with green space near most neighborhoods, 72 percent of people sixty and older reported not having used a park in the previous year. An Age-Friendly Parks Checklist was created, so that park managers and users could evaluate what improvements needed to be made—things like shady areas and paths; public toilets that are accessible and clean; signs with large, clear lettering; and a variety of programs to engage people of all ages.

For the healthy eating goal, Philadelphia is going far beyond the traditional lunch at a senior center and meals-on-wheels. A Healthy Cart Program brings fresh produce, low-fat dairy, and whole grain products to low-income neighborhoods. Throughout the city, intergenerational community gardens are being planted, many with accessible raised beds. One church donated space for three joined gardens especially for older adults, built by volunteers of all ages who donated a thousand hours of time. "Seniors plant, harvest, and cook the produce, both at the [seniors] center and at home, and will soon be selling it at a nearby farmers' market," according to the report.

In all these initiatives, communities connect with ongoing programs, partner with a wide range of community groups, and chart a roadmap to a future that includes a much higher portion of older people.

CHAPTER 13

How Will We Pay?
Planning for the Unknown

Underlying the hopeful alternatives in this book are significant questions of who will pay for services that people may need in order to remain out of institutions. Those who say they wish to age in place (unless that place is a continuing care retirement community which includes long-term care) need to consider how they will pay for major adaptations to their home or for help if they need it. Such help may be for mopping floors, mowing the lawn, or bathing, or it may be for transportation when we can no longer drive. If we become truly debilitated we will need to pay for in-home care, which, at $20 an hour, can quickly soak up resources. Perhaps nothing reflects our mass denial about aging more than our refusal to contemplate ahead of time how to pay for help when we need it. Without a plan, aging in place may be nothing more than wishful thinking.

The public remains woefully ignorant about such matters. The results of a 2009 MetLife survey were typical. Two-thirds of respondents did not know how nursing homes, assisted living, and home care are paid for; they assumed that Medicare, private health insurance, or disability insurance paid for such services. They do not, and they never have. (Medicare only pays for some short-term stays in nursing homes.) "A wide range of the population ages 40–70 is unaware of its potential need for care and how to pay for it. Most are not taking appropriate steps to protect themselves from potentially catastrophic expenses," according to the survey.[1]

Despite what everyone knows is a burgeoning need, the government has no plans to expand Medicare to encompass long-term care. A modest long-term care benefit of $50 a day, known as the CLASS Act, was proposed as part of the Affordable Care Act. But that was eliminated early on, in part because of partisanship, but as importantly, because the program as designed was not sustainable.

It's no great mystery how to cover people's long-term care needs. Other countries have done it for decades. In much of Europe, for example, home care for older people is a matter of course, not some mountain each family must climb alone. As Sara Mansfield Taber wrote in her essay, "Caring for Mom, Mum and Maman," the difference between how the United States handles eldercare contrasts sharply with that provided in Great Britain and France.[2] Sara's mother paid $4,000 a month for assisted living. On top of that, her mother hired private aides for an additional $1,400 a month because she needed more care than could be provided by the staff on her floor, where a single aide had to care for thirty-eight people. In contrast, her friend Fiona's "mum," Pat, in England, had terrible pain from diabetes and arthritis but she received considerable public support. "A government-supplied home health aide visits Pat at breakfast, lunch and dinner every day. This costs the family 120 pounds a week (approximately $785 per month), a little more than half of what my mom paid for private aides." And of course, the British family was able to keep "Mum" at home, where she wanted to be, because of the generous support.

Meanwhile, in France, Sara's friend Juliette also took care of her *maman*, Madelaine, at her mother's home. Her mother, who has Alzheimer's disease, is assisted through a government program for older and disabled people called the "Personal Autonomy Allocation." "Since the government refunds 560 of every 1,200 euros Juliette spends on her mother's medical expenses, she is able to hire a caregiver who looks after her mother around the clock 3½ days per week. This allows Madelaine to stay in her suburban Paris home, where her family has lived for three generations, and provides Juliette a regular respite from elder care," she wrote.

The odds of programs like this being enacted in the United States are long, to say the least. In our country, the primary federal-state program that does help pay for long-term care is Medicaid, the insurance program for low-income people or people who have spent down most of their assets. Indeed, older people in nursing homes consume an enormous chunk of the Medicaid budget—nearly one-third in 2012. Or, put another way, Medicaid is the primary payer for nearly two-thirds of all nursing home residents.[3] These funds also must cover children living in poverty, the working poor, and the unemployed. The Affordable Care Act adds to the pool of Medicaid beneficiaries by raising income eligibility.

For decades, federal and state funding for long-term care through Medicaid has been skewed toward nursing homes, never mind what older people actually wanted. Many people ended up in nursing homes for the simple reason that they ran out of money, and Medicaid was mandated only to pay for a nursing home, not for assisted living or home care, even if these options were less expensive. This has been changing as states shift more funds to home- and community-based services in a process called "rebalancing" (not that it was ever balanced). Still, in 2009, 55 percent of Medicaid's long-term care (LTC) dollars went to people in nursing homes, even though this group represented only 38 percent of the people receiving Medicaid long-term care benefits. Moreover, despite home- and community-based services costing less, "36 states spent a majority of their Medicaid LTC dollars on institutional care, and only 12 states and Washington, DC, spent half or more of their LTC dollars on [home- and community-based services] in 2009."[4]

"Words like 'choice' and 'self-determination,' 'consumer preferences' and 'quality of life' are becoming a more natural part of the conversation when policymakers and providers discuss long-term service and support options. Yet providers, health experts and lawmakers have not yet been successful in translating these ideals into policy and funding decisions that affect the day-to-day delivery of care in a meaningful way for the majority of the elderly," according to a report by Leading Age (formerly the American Association of Health and Services for the Aging), the trade association representing nonprofit long-term care providers.[5] The report notes the fragmented and confusing "system" that confronts people seeking to access services that would allow them to remain in their own homes.

For middle class people, counting on the government as their default for meeting long-term care needs may not be a reasonable strategy—at least not if their goal is to avoid a nursing home. A study by the National Institute on Aging found that if states doubled the amount of money they spend on home- and community-based services, they could reduce by 35 percent the chance that an older person without children would wind up in a nursing home. Yet states are cutting back rather than investing more in such services.[6]

No doubt some believe that the government doesn't have any business helping families with long-term care costs anyway. How viable, then, are private pay options for most Americans? A report by the AARP Public Policy Institute sums it up succinctly: "Private pay nursing home care is not affordable for middle-income families anywhere. While less costly than nursing homes, home health care is still unaffordable for middle-income older people at typical levels of use."[7]

Moreover, the AARP report found considerable variation among states as far as affordability, with some of the higher-income states being the most affordable as far as home care while people in poorer states are paying more due to lack of competition. Among other strategies for promoting affordable services, the report suggests more support for family caregivers, through respite care, education and training, as well as family leave and flextime for working caregivers. But states seem in no mood to expand services, even if it would lead to more people being able to pay for care themselves.

Of course millions of fortunate elders have another option: family members willing and able to assist them. Family caregivers contributed the equivalent of $450 billion in 2009, according to another study by the AARP Public Policy Institute. To help us wrap our minds around this figure, AARP offers some helpful comparisons: $450 billion is nearly four times Medicaid spending in 2009 on long-term care services ($119 billion). It's more than the total global sales of Wal-Mart ($408 billion in 2009), and nearly as much as the total funding for Medicare that year.[8]

Family caregivers often sacrifice their own career advancement, sick leave, and vacations, or even quit their jobs in order to take care of their parents or spouse. A strong body of literature has shown that family caregivers, even as they have deep feelings of satisfaction in helping their loved ones, are often stressed out and suffer their own medical and emotional problems as a result of their caregiving burdens. The amount of paid in-home help has been *declining* since the mid-1990s, "and more family caregivers today are left to carry the load alone."[9]

For a quick primer on the messy finances of paying for long-term care, I called Howard Gleckman, resident fellow at the Urban Institute and author of *Caring for Our Parents: Inspiring Stories of Families Seeking New Solutions to America's Most Urgent Health Care Crisis*. Since most everyone says they want to "age in place," I asked him, how will we pay for it?

"The short answer is," he said, "we have no idea."

Long-Term Care Insurance

For decades, we have been told that a prudent person would purchase long-term care insurance to cover the potential costs of home care, assisted living, or nursing home. But the portion of people buying this insurance has remained stuck at around seven percent, at most. In recent years, many insurers have thrown in the towel. MetLife and Prudential are among the giants that have pulled out of the market, "because their actuarial assumptions regarding the viability of the product had been too optimistic."[10] (These companies continue to honor long-term care insurance policies already purchased.)

"The private long-term care insurance industry is imploding," said Howard. "It's completely falling apart."

Perhaps 200,000 new individual policies were sold in 2012, at a time when you'd expect baby boomers might be considering purchasing such a product. But a combination of factors has discouraged consumers from buying long-term care insurance.

For one, the price can seem high. The national average is $2,283 a year, and increases the later you wait to purchase it. For example, those younger than fifty-five pay an average of $1,831 in annual premiums, while those seventy-five and older pay $4,123.[11] You typically pay those premiums as long as you don't need the benefits—potentially forever. Many options affect the price, including the dollar amount of the daily benefit you wish to purchase, whether the policy includes a protection against inflation, how many years of benefits and how big a deductible you want, meaning do you want the benefits to kick in immediately or not for thirty, sixty, or ninety days. Many preexisting conditions and any hint of dementia will likely prevent you from getting coverage.

In addition to the expense, many consumers cite mistrust of insurance companies to actually come through for them and concern about potential rate increases. Horror stories in the media contribute to these worries. One recent *New York Times* story told of a woman, seventy-four, who had suffered a serious stroke and was left with "the problem-solving and safety awareness equal to a 6-year-old." She could no longer live safely on her own and her family had moved her to assisted living. They had tried for five months to get her long-term care insurance to start paying benefits but had gotten nowhere. Only with the intervention of the *Times* reporter, who writes a consumer-advocate column, were they helped.[12]

Such fears may be overblown. A 2008 survey by the US Department of Health and Human Services found that 94 percent of long-term care insurance claimants were satisfied after having made a claim.[13] Nevertheless, worrisome news stories can stick with the public. Moreover, our old friend Denial no doubt also plays a role. For years, surveys have shown that roughly one-third of respondents think they will ever need long-term care,[14] despite being told that 70 percent of those over sixty-five will at some point.[15]

From the insurers' point of view, Howard explained, long-term care insurance as a business model fell apart during the recession with its stubbornly-low interest rates. "The biggest problem has nothing to do with lack of demand and high prices, it's all about interest rates," he said. The original idea was that consumers would buy long-term care insurance when they were fifty, pay the premiums for thirty years, then collect the benefits, if needed, in their eighties. Insurers would make money off the interest from the premiums during those decades. But with interest rates at near zero, coupled with the requirement that companies invest the money in low-risk products such as bonds, it doesn't add up. "This is a particular problem when most long-term care policies come with inflation protection of five percent compounded interest," he added. "If you're earning one percent but your liability is increasing five percent a year, you're going to get killed."

Those consumers who tried to be responsible and purchase long-term care insurance have been rewarded in many cases with steep rate increases. Some insurers charge periodic rate increases of 40 to 50 percent, raise premiums for women (who live longer), get rid of a spousal discount, or tighten underwriting standards—none of which endear them to more consumers.

The emerging field of genetic testing may be the nail in the coffin for long-term care insurance as we've known it. On the near horizon, people may learn through genetic testing what their prospects are for getting all sorts of disease, including Alzheimer's. As it stands now, long-term care insurers—unlike health insurers, thanks to the Affordable Care Act—are allowed to discriminate against people who are predisposed to an expensive condition or illness by denying them coverage or charging them exorbitant rates.

Even if that law were to be changed, and such discrimination were banned, long-term care insurers would have no choice but to assume that any policyholder was a potential Alzheimer's patient and charge them accordingly. After all, half of those consumers now paying long-term care insurance premiums actually do get dementia, so it's not surprising that insurers want to protect themselves.

Some experts maintain hope that consumers will wise up and start purchasing long-term care insurance, despite the challenges. "A large untapped market potential remains for long-term care insurance, but many educational and attitudinal factors need to be overcome," according to one scholarly article. "Although long-term care insurance is neither feasible nor suitable for everyone, among those who have considered the purchase and chosen not to buy, the majority are still considering it as a viable option."[16]

Others have come up with strategies for changing long-term care insurance in ways to make it more affordable, such as high-deductible policies with consumers paying the first two years of care, annual premium indexing to avoid big rate hikes, or tax credits to encourage middle-income consumers to purchase long-term care insurance.

With traditional long-term care insurance on the ropes, insurers are coming up with new products that may appeal to people with the means to pay for them. So-called "combo" products combine annuities or life insurance with long-term care insurance. A $200,000 life insurance policy, say, could be tapped for long-term care needs, or an annuity might pay only a modest benefit when you're in your sixties, but a more generous one when you hit your eighties.

What about reverse mortgages or home equity loans? For those who survived the recession and housing crisis with value still left in their homes, they may be able to tap into some of their property's worth. Reverse mortgages allow homeowners to turn their home equity into cash, without paying interest. Like long-term care insurance, there have been considerable fluctuations in reverse mortgages. Some elders purchased products that were unsound or used the money up so rapidly they ended up at risk of losing their home, unable to pay insurance and property taxes.

Still, AARP found that most people who have reverse mortgages have been satisfied, and with no great option on the horizon, many of us will likely turn to the value in our home to help pay for care. According to an article in *Public Policy & Aging Report*, "The next big driver of the reverse mortgage market could be out-of-pocket health and long-term care costs. Boomers will need resources for aging in place as health care is being shifted into the home, with earlier hospital discharges and already overburdened family caregivers handling complex medical procedures."[17]

Howard Gleckman and others suggest that linking health care to long-term care may make sense, both financially and in giving people what they want. Howard offers a common scenario of an eighty-year-old woman with congestive heart failure (CHF) who lives at home and participates in a managed care plan that covers all her medical needs and long-term care for a set monthly fee. He said,

> You can either pay for her repeated trips to the hospital, or you can say we'll pay for modest levels of assistance at home that might do a lot to keep her out of the hospital. One of the key issues with CHF is weighing somebody regularly. Maybe you have a digitally hooked up scale, or maybe an aide who comes in a few hours a day, and checks the weight. Maybe that aide can help with diet, maybe you've got somebody who can arrange for transportation to get [the patient] to the doctor or she may have arthritis and you can help her get to physical therapy. There's a whole package of relatively inexpensive interventions that could improve quality of life and reduce health care costs, but aren't what we normally think of as benefits you receive from long-term care insurance or from Medicaid. It's an argument that I find pretty attractive.

In fact, he said, the state of Florida is trying something similar, paying a managed care company $500 per month per patient for those who are "dual-eligibles," meaning they are on both Medicare and Medicaid.

Howard concluded,

The story here is the system we have now is not working. It's not sustainable. We're really going to have to think of much more creative ways to do this. It's probably going to include some private insurance—welfare-based Medicaid is not the way to do it. I would do it through Medicare, but that's probably not possible politically. We all want to get care at home, but there's got to be some way to pay for it and we just don't have that all figured out.

CHAPTER 14

Who Will Help Us?
Advocating for Direct Care Workers

As Howard Gleckman and other experts suggest, remaining in our own homes as we age ultimately becomes a health care issue. If we're healthy, the odds are decent we can age in place if we wish. But if we have problems, we need to come to grips with the fact that there are simply not enough paid caregivers in the pipeline to assist us. Even for those lucky enough to have the financial resources to pay for in-home care, it will grow ever more difficult to find competent, caring help. Whether it's home care aides, visiting nurses, or physicians who make house calls, we need a concerted effort to entice more professionals to the geriatrics field, or it will be impossible for many people to stay in their own communities as they wish.

In 2011 there were already some 2.5 million home health aides, who assist people with hands-on care, checking vital signs, skin care, exercise, and medication, and personal care aides, who help with housekeeping, cooking, and companionship but do not provide health care. The majority of these workers are employed by an agency; the rest are hired directly by the client.[1]

According to the Bureau of Labor Statistics (BLS) *Occupational Outlook Handbook*, the ranks of home health aides and personal care aides will swell by 70 percent from 2010 to 2020[2]—and that's before the baby boomers hit their most frail years. That figure compares to a 14 percent projection for all jobs over the decade. In its good news–bad news outlook, BLS notes: "Job prospects for both home health aides and personal care aides are excellent. These occupations are large and expected to grow very quickly, thus adding many jobs. In addition, the low pay and high emotional demands cause many workers to leave these occupations, and they will have to be replaced."

How their ranks will not only be replaced but expanded is left dangling, a mystery yet to be solved. The message to those with a fondness for older people and a desire to serve continues to be: We need you! We promise you a job! We'll pay you miserly wages and put you through the wringer! Join us!

The late Leonila Vega, executive director of the New York–based Direct Care Alliance (DCA), a worker advocacy organization, talked with me in 2010 about our society's lack of understanding and preparation for the growing numbers of frail elders wanting to age in place. "People want to stay independent as long as they can," she said. "There's a misperception that home care workers help clean, shop, other light activities. That's true, they do those things, but they're caring for older clients with more complex conditions, multiple chronic care issues, and [the clients] are staying in the home with a lot more complicated care plans. [Direct care workers] are the ones who have to keep this person safe."

The job can be both difficult and gratifying. On the one hand, aides have a sense of real purpose. They take pride and satisfaction in their important role as caregiver and companion to those who are old or disabled. "It's one of the most rewarding jobs I've ever had," Tracy Dudzinski, a long-time home health aide and a leader of Cooperative Care in Wautoma, Wisconsin, a worker's co-op, told me, "to go in and the person is so happy to see you. You're the only person they're going to see that day. I call it feeding my need."

Yet the job is tough. Aides, who are often hired by adult children, may be resented or only grudgingly accepted by the client. As BLS describes it:

Home health and personal care aides had a higher-than-average number of work-related injuries and illnesses in 2010. Work as an aide can be physically and emotionally demanding. Aides must guard against back injury because they may have to move clients into and out of bed or help them to stand or walk.

In addition, aides may frequently work with clients who have cognitive impairments or mental health issues and who may display difficult or violent behaviors. Aides may also face hazards from minor infections and exposure to communicable diseases.[3]

Moreover even as they toil to help people who have serious medical conditions or disabilities, the aides themselves frequently lack health insurance or other benefits, such as paid time off for sickness or vacation. Astonishingly, until recently, they have not been covered by basic labor protections, such as the minimum wage or mandatory time-and-a-half pay for working more than forty hours a week. "There's no other industry that is comparable in size and importance that says it's basically okay to not pay overtime and exempt people from minimum wage protection," Leonila Vega said. "It's absolutely unconscionable."

President Barack Obama agreed. At a 2011 press conference, where he announced he was directing the Department of Labor to address this inequity, he said, "As the home care business has changed over the years, the law hasn't changed to keep up . . . that means these workers are lumped together with teenage babysitters. You can wake up at five thirty in the morning and take the late bus home at night and still not make the minimum wage. That's just wrong. And in this country it's inexcusable."

That action must be taken by the President of the United States to ensure direct care workers earn the minimum wage boggles the mind. The "law" of supply and demand would suggest that dangerous jobs in such high demand would command decent wages. But because neither the government nor the public feel they can afford paying a living wage, direct care workers are left to subsidize home care for the rest of us through their paltry pay. According to the Paraprofessional Healthcare Institute (PHI), nearly half the direct-care workforce can only get part-time work, thus lowering their annual earnings even more.[4]

Susan Misiorski, director of PHI's coaching and consulting services, explained,

> On the home care side, getting consistent hours is difficult. If you're on a case and it's supposed to be eight hours a day, forty hours a week, and if that person goes into the hospital, you're down hours. If that person passes away, it can take a while before a new case is given to you to replace those hours. It may not be an eight-hour case—it can be a two-hour case. Being able to anticipate the consistent paycheck in home- and community-based services is a real challenge. The other huge challenge is transportation, if you're in an environment that doesn't have a good public transportation system and you need to travel in a car and you're making $8 an hour. Many home care agencies do not pay you while you're driving—they'll reimburse your mileage. If I have a two-hour case with Mrs. Jones and then I need to leave for another one- or two-hour case, I'm off the clock between their homes. That's true in most organizations.

From 2001 to 2011, home care workers actually *lost* ground, with their inflation-adjusted wages declining by 12 percent during that time. In 2011, home health aides averaged $9.91 an hour, and personal care aides earned $9.49.[5]

That's how much society values the work of those who care for our frailest, most vulnerable elders—our grandparents and parents—who need help to remain in their own homes. (And it's not much better for those who work in assisted living and nursing homes.) It's a shameful and stark reflection of the lack of support not only for these workers but for families. Even if families want to do the right thing, they may simply not have the resources to pay a living wage and benefits. (Families have to pay far more to a home health agency per hour than an aide receives.) At the same time there is often a mismatch between client and caregiver needs. An older person may only need an hour or two of care a day or even less, while an aide needs a full-time job.

It's no coincidence that the ranks of direct care workers are filled by women, many of them single mothers, African Americans, and immigrants, of whom one in five is estimated to be undocumented. Most of the immigrant direct-care workforce is concentrated in twenty-four metropolitan areas, such as the greater Miami area, where 74 percent of direct care workers are foreign-born, and New York City where 66 percent of direct care workers are.[6]

In addition to difficult working conditions and lousy pay, direct care workers are typically not given adequate training. Here again, there is a lack of investment in people to whom we entrust those with complex medical or cognitive problems. To be compensated through Medicare or Medicaid, nurse's aides need only seventy-five hours' worth of training (some states require more). Personal care aides are generally not covered by insurance and no training is required. Advocates for direct care workers are fond of pointing out that cosmetologists are required to have far more training to become licensed, typically a nine-month program.

Peggy Powell, national director of curriculum and workforce development for PHI, stresses that training is fundamental to both good jobs and good care. But as a society we have not invested in it. "Because everyone is figuring how to make more with less, they'll cut education and training to the barest minimum," she said of home health agencies. "Our position is that if you invest in training you'll have less turnover." This helps everyone.

With as many as five million people with Alzheimer's disease and many more projected to have cognitive loss as the population ages, Peggy Powell said there's a particular need for dementia-care training. She describes the intense pressure home care workers are under as families worry about their loved ones' safety.

The home care worker is on the front line to constantly ensure [their clients] are safe, with little training and support of how to do this and how to address the challenges that come up. How do you de-escalate when someone is agitated? How do you not unintentionally contribute to that agitation? How do you begin to read the person, to observe the person, to intervene at earlier parts before they become agitated? It cannot be done through reading and PowerPoint presentations. It cannot be done in one two-week session. [The aide] needs to be introduced to a body of knowledge, skills, and attitudes that are important, and they need their own support system.

Her sentiments were echoed in a 2008 Institute of Medicine report on the need to beef up the health care workforce for an aging America. As far as training of aides, "The committee concluded that current federal training minimums are inadequate to prepare direct-care workers and that the content of the training lacks sufficient geriatric-specific content."[7] It noted that while people are remaining at home with increasingly complex medical problems, the required number of hours of training has not changed since 1987. The report did not mince words in its conclusion: "The future health care workforce will be woefully inadequate in its capacity to meet the large demand for health services for older adults if current patterns of care and of the training of providers continue."[8]

Again, such training and skills-building are not rocket science. There is a large body of knowledge and many highly developed training programs available. The problem is a lack of commitment to investing in it.

One modest step was made through the Affordable Care Act, which awarded $5 million in three-year grants to six states—California, Iowa, Michigan, Massachusetts, Maine, and North Carolina—to develop and strengthen their training for direct-care workers, with an aim toward expanding and improving the workforce. The states' final reports were expected at the end of 2013, with the hope that strategies and lessons learned would be transferrable to other states wishing to expand their direct-care workforce.

Despite the well-recognized and looming need for direct-care workers and for a way to pay them, Congress has not acted to address the issue.

Taking matters into their own hands, direct care workers and their supporters are working on several fronts to gain more respect and hopefully higher wages.

- In 1985, Cooperative Home Care Associates was organized in the Bronx as a worker-owned business to improve working conditions and training. It began with a dozen home health aides and now has two thousand. To improve their members' training, the cooperative partnered with PHI. A similar co-op, Home Care Associates, was organized in Philadelphia.
- In Wautoma, Wisconsin, home care workers formed a cooperative in 2001 called Cooperative Care. Their goal is to earn more respect and to provide their members with better pay, benefits, and a career path upward. Even with the co-op, Tracy Dudzinski said, "Our workers live paycheck to paycheck and sometimes it doesn't even stretch."

   What the co-op has given its members are opportunities for leadership development and a voice in their work lives. The co-op began its own training and mentoring program to improve skills. Tracy has also stretched her wings by becoming active in the DCA and has had the opportunity to testify in Washington on Capitol Hill and at the Department of Labor on behalf of direct care workers.

- DCA lobbied at the national level for wage protections for home care workers that would put them in line with the rest of the American workforce, as directed by President Obama in 2011. The rule sat for more than a year following the public comment period. More than twenty thousand people commented, most of them reportedly in support of direct care workers.

Finally, on September 17, 2013, home care workers won the right to be protected under the Fair Labor Standards Act. In 2015 the law is to take effect. At this writing, some in Congress were seeking to undermine the act.

Other efforts are focused on bringing nurses and physicians to frail elders' homes. House calls, once commonplace, all but disappeared from the US health care system in the twentieth century. Community nursing, once a key piece of health care delivery, was often cut. But today a small but growing number of health care providers, including physicians, are willing to visit homebound patients.

A 2011 article in the journal *American Family Physician* noted that seeing patients in their home environment gives doctors a window to provide better care. "House calls can provide a unique perspective on a patient's life that is not available in an office visit or during hospitalization," the article noted. "A house call can foster the physician-patient relationship, and enhance the physician's understanding of the patient's environment and support systems."[9]

Although the authors found that research on the outcomes of home visits was mixed, the results of several studies were promising. Among veterans receiving home care from a multidisciplinary team, for example, patients had fewer hospital admissions and readmissions, shorter lengths of stay, and a reduction in long-term care facility stays.

Katie McDonough, a social worker and executive director of Capitol Hill Village, said CHV's most vulnerable members have benefited greatly from a Medical House Calls Program. Visits by a multidisciplinary team in the member's home is far better than a visit to the doctor's office, Katie said. "For long-term care and for care of frail older adults who are living in the community, a typical primary care model isn't enough. I don't care how good the doctor is. It's just not enough to address the needs they have."

More recently, with pressure from the Centers for Medicare and Medicaid

Services to reduce hospital readmissions, some providers are increasing their home care services. A "Hospital at Home" program in Albuquerque diverts patients who would have been admitted from the emergency room, sending them back home where they are followed with intensive services. A study of Hospital at Home found that not only were patients more satisfied and their clinical outcomes comparable or better, but costs were 19 percent lower compared to similar patients who had been admitted to the hospital.[10]

The Affordable Care Act included an Independence At Home demonstration project to see if care delivered by doctors and nurse practitioners to patients' homes will lead to higher quality care at a more affordable cost. The program is aimed at elders who are on traditional Medicare and who meet particular eligibility requirements, such as having two or more chronic conditions, needing help with two or more activities of daily living, and having been admitted to the hospital and to rehabilitation during the previous year. Eighteen providers around the nation were chosen for the demonstration, which is underway at this writing.

Another promising program is the Department of Veterans Affair's medical foster home program. Veterans, who might otherwise have to move to a nursing home, live with a family unrelated to them, who are trained to provide basic care as well as meals, housekeeping, and transportation. The caregivers are connected with VA nurses through a telehealth monitoring system to stay on top of problems. The veterans pay the families directly, from $1,500 to $3,000 a month depending on their needs, usually relying on their military pensions and Social Security. Again, this is far less costly and more appealing to many frail veterans. The program has been expanded to sites in most states.

In programs such as this, the caregiving workforce is augmented by people in the community. The federal Cash and Counseling program, for example, encourages those on Medicaid to direct their own home care and allows them to hire relatives or friends. The hope is not only that older people will benefit from more control of their care, but that the home care workforce can be increased in an informal way. The first Cash and Counseling demonstration project was Arkansas's Independent Choices. It found that consumers were significantly more satisfied than those who received the traditional regulated agency care.[11] The home care workers too were satisfied. In a study comparing related home care workers with agency workers who had been hired directly by consumers, both groups reported high levels of satisfaction, despite low pay and lack of benefits. (Those who were related to the consumer, however, were more likely than agency workers to report emotional strain.) Most of the workers hired directly enjoyed a close relationship with the consumer and appreciated the flexible hours.

Arkansas made Independent Choices a permanent program, and many other states are now experimenting with what is called "consumer-directed care" for their Medicaid population. This could be a promising avenue for low-income elders who wish to age in place but need assistance.

Only through creative responses such as these will we be able to support all of those who wish to remain in their own communities. The answer for most people may be to use a combination of savings and home equity to pay for help, along with informal support from family, neighbors, friends, congregation members, and volunteers to help fill the gap—which might be a good thing. The pool of potential helpers is free of course. But more importantly, this is exactly what the architects of many of the alternatives in this book are doing. This solution is rooted in relationship. It potentially transforms long-term care from an unsustainable program that treats elders as passive recipients of services to a normal life stage that draws on elders' own strengths and support systems to piece together a life at home that works, one that is based on reciprocity and meaning.

CHAPTER 15

Is There a Robot in Your Future?
Accepting Non-Human Help

In the 2012 film *Robot & Frank*, an aging cat burglar, played by the veteran actor Frank Langella, finds support and friendship with a shiny white robot that his son bought him as a caregiver.[1] Frank had developed serious memory problems, his home was a mess, and he was subsisting on Cap'n Crunch. He refused to move to "the memory center," so to his son, the robot seemed the next best thing.

"You have got to be kidding," says the incredulous Frank when he first sees the robot. "I am not this pathetic. I don't have to be spoon-fed by some God-damn robot."

When his son tries to convince him the robot is more like "a butler," Frank responds, "That thing is going to murder me in my sleep."

But Robot (Frank refuses to name it) is here to stay. It has been programmed to keep Frank healthy and is a gourmet health cook. So long sweet cereal, hello kale. Robot encourages Frank to get off his duff, take long walks, and "find a hobby." Before long, Frank's brilliant idea for a hobby is to train Robot to assist him in his next heist.

The film, set in "the near future," gives other glimpses of what may soon await us. When Frank receives a telephone call at home, he doesn't have to pick up a receiver. A disembodied voice tells him who is calling and if he wishes to talk, he simply says hello and the image of the caller (usually one of his two children) appears on a large screen. When he visits his beloved library, his favorite librarian (played by Susan Sarandan) tells him dejectedly they are closing for "renovation"—meaning getting rid of their last books and creating instead an "environment." We hear the obnoxious "library environment" consultant discuss a planned historical display about the Dewey Decimal system.

Most poignant though is Frank's growing relationship with Robot as it becomes a pal as well as an accomplice. Although Robot is not meant to have moral and ethical agency, we can easily imagine how emotionally tied one could become to this walking, talking machine that is willing to sacrifice itself for Frank's well-being.

As someone who is a bit of a Luddite myself, the film challenged me to wonder "Why not?" Since few in our society have either the interest (the government and the private sector) or the means (most of the public) to pay real, live, home care workers a living wage, why not seek help from a robotic friend?

I took a trip to Atlanta to discuss the future of robotics and home technology with researchers at Georgia Institute of Technology, who are leaders in studying cutting-edge ways to help older adults remain in their homes.

At the Human Factors and Aging Lab (human factors is an emerging branch of psychology dealing with how people interact with products, physical environments, and equipment or technology), researchers conducted in-depth interviews with twenty-one people aged sixty-five to ninety-three about their views of receiving help from a robot. Participants were first shown a video of Honda's robot "Asimo," and then given a checklist of forty-eight tasks. They were asked, "Imagine you needed help with this task. Would you prefer a human or a robot?"

"What was really impressive to me was how open-minded the older adults were to robot assistance," said professor Wendy Rogers, co-director of the lab. For many tasks, participants had no preference for a human over a robot, and in fact for some tasks they actually preferred a robot—including for housekeeping, laundry, medication reminders, learning something new, and hobbies. Conversely, on average, participants reported they would prefer human assistance for more personal tasks such as bathing and dressing; preparing meals and deciding on which medication; and helping with social interaction, such as entertaining.[2]

Another surprising finding, said Jenay Beer, who was completing her doctoral work there, is that older adults like the idea of "collaborating" with a robot, rather than just sitting there ordering the robot around. For example, a robot might be useful for pulling the troublesome bottom fitted sheet on a mattress, while the older person would complete the task of changing the top sheet and blankets. "The big goal for the older adults was to keep doing what they could," added Cory-Ann Smarr, whose dissertation focuses on understanding whether and how older people will accept robots in their homes.

It also became clear that customizing what the robot did for the particular person would be important. Going to Best Buy and buying a robot off the shelf that can adapt to your house and your needs is a long way off.

From the Human Factors and Aging Lab, Jenay and I headed across the campus to another novel facility at Georgia Tech, the Aware Home. This lovely 5,000-plus-square-foot three-story house was built as a research lab in 2000, to give researchers a way to study new technologies in a home environment. Older people who wish to participate in research come to the house to try out new monitoring and sensing systems. There I met Hai Nguyen, who was finishing up his doctoral work at Georgia Tech's Healthcare Robotics Lab, and GATSBII (pronounced Gatsby), a full-size robot. GATSBII is a PR2 assistive robot, created by Willow Garage in Menlo Park, California, to give researchers like those at Georgia Tech a way to experiment with how robots might help older adults or people with disabilities. PR2 is known as a "mobile manipulator," meaning it can both move across the floor and manipulate its hands.

GATSBII looks more like a gigantic Transformer toy than a human. It stands more than five feet five inches on a base the size of a large wheelchair and weighs four hundred pounds, the size of an adult gorilla. Its arms are immense, but through specially designed shoulders that bear much of the weight, the arms feel light and easy for a small woman like me to move.[3]

"PR2 was way too big for the older adults we showed it to," Jenay told me. "There was concern about it damaging knick-knacks." People do not want a robot so large it feels intimidating, the researchers learned, so future robots will be trimmer. Size is one of many challenges. The robot needs to be able to reach high up on a shelf to, say, retrieve a bowl or low enough to pick up a thimble under a footstool. To achieve both, the PR2 has a telescoping spine that allows it to grow and shrink on command.

Generally, older people who have met GATSBII were excited and curious. "Many older adults felt more positive after the exposure to the robot," said Jenay. "Exposure matters."

In her research, graduate student Akanksha Prakash studied whether older people would prefer that robots looked more human or more machine-like. Just over half preferred a more human-looking robot. "When I asked them why would they prefer a human face," she said, "one of the prime reasons was familiarity, and that's what many roboticists claim because humans are hardwired for human interaction. That would ease and enhance the quality of interaction. However people were attributing a lot of human-like qualities onto this appearance. Some said, 'I would find this robot to be a companion or more capable.'"

The first non-human assistants for older people or those with disabilities were not robots but animals, Hai explained, specifically monkeys and dogs. Both could be trained to fetch objects, and monkeys, with their amazingly dexterous hands, can perform all sorts of tasks, such as inserting a DVD in a player, putting a drinking straw in a cup, and gently scratching an itch on someone's face. When researchers first began developing assistive robots, they realized that emulating monkeys would be daunting, so they began with tasks such as fetching socks and opening doors and drawers.

"One of the arguments against robots was you could install motors and sensors in the home to do much the same thing," Hai said. "But instead of having to install motors in every door and drawer and light switch, you're squeezing all that into a robot." Plus, a robot potentially could go outside your home, assisting you with grocery shopping, for example.

One early attempt at robotic companions was a fake dog in a nursing home setting. In one eight-week study, the Sony version, "Aibo," was found to ease loneliness in nursing home residents as well as a real pooch did.[4] Another study of nursing home residents with dementia found that a robotic animal "yielded significantly longer engagement durations, more attention, and a more positive attitude" than did a plush animal. Moreover, participants were at least as engaged with a robotic dog as a real dog.[5] (But, not as engaged as with a real baby, I was relieved to learn.)

As for household chores, for years simpler robots such as the Roomba have been available for consumers to use as vacuum cleaners. The robots of tomorrow are expected to be far more sophisticated and able to engage in conversation. In Japan, the robot called Twenty-One—which doesn't look terribly different from the cinematic robot friend of Frank—can pick up a straw, stick it in a glass, and hand it to a person. Other human-size robots can tend bar or even play the violin. The young research team at Willow Garage trained PR2 to fetch a Guinness from the fridge—it will even open the bottle if you don't have a church key handy.

When I arrived at the Aware Home, Hai had just been working with GATSBII to teach it to turn a light switch on and off. Hai demonstrated the robot's success. While not speedy—the task took ninety-five seconds from when Hai clicked on his computer to give the command—the robot indeed turned off the light. The scratches on the wall were evidence of the trial-and-error nature of the training. "It collects experiences," said Hai. "It stores an image of the location and the effect. When it gets to the light switch, it knows something happened. To the robot, the light switch is defined by its effects—it changed the level of brightness, which the robot sensed."

A robot's "eyes" are basically a camera, so detecting light is relatively simple. Although, Hai noted, if a bright ray of sunlight pierced through the venetian blinds and fell on the light switch, "It might confuse the robot."

The robot has a repertoire of behaviors it has learned, such as tracking people, opening doors and drawers, and grabbing objects as delicate as an egg or a light bulb in its pincer-hands. It can even play pool or give a rudimentary "massage." (Having experienced the robot's pincers on my back, I don't think massage therapists have much to fear.) To teach it to open a refrigerator, Hai can take the robot's arm and train it how to complete the task. But, he explained, the robot will need to know things like, "Where on the fridge should I grab?" "Does it matter where my elbow is?

"It exactly copies the motion, but you want a more generalized behavior," Hai said. "You can teach it that it doesn't matter where [its] elbow is."

Robots also can take on the personality of the person who trained it. Thus their actions may reflect if they've been taught by a careful, cautious person or a more reckless Devil-may-care sort.

Today the PR2 is for research institutions and far too costly for consumers—about $400,000. But Hai hopes that in the not too distant future the cost for an assistive robot could come down to $5,000 to $10,000.

He imagines himself with a robot that would be at home, waiting for Hai's instructions that he'd arrive in thirty minutes. The robot would open the refrigerator, take out a chicken that was in a pan, and put it in the oven. The robot would have picked up the house and watered the plants while Hai was gone, and greet him at the door when he returned. Unlike Robot in the film, Hai thinks we've got a ways to go before a home robot would prepare elaborate meals or act as a companion.

The uniqueness of each home and the need for customization makes personal robots especially difficult to develop, explained research scientists Matei Ciocarlie and Kaijen Hsiao of Willow Garage, who head up the team that created PR2. They envision robots being an important aid to help older people remain independent in their own homes or to assist human caregivers.

"Robotic technology and in particular mobile manipulation can be a solution to the aging population problem and the shortage of care workers that we face now and will be facing in the future," Matei told me in a phone interview.

> We just won't have enough care workers in the next twenty years. Care workers are going to be stretched too thin so we're hoping robotic technology can help with that quite significantly in terms of reducing the number of chores and menial tasks—things like getting supplies, moving things around, simple chores—so that a caregiver can actually focus on providing care. If you talk to caregivers, they say they would like help with all kinds of tasks that have nothing to do with their vocation as caregivers. We're hoping robotic technology, far from replacing caregivers, rather allows them to focus on what they're best at and what they enjoy doing.

Kaijen added that the robot could help out in the middle of the night, when a caregiver might not be there. "If the person drops something and can't get it, the caregiver could log in remotely and teleoperate the robot to help the person," she said.

The researchers have been helped tremendously by the participation of Henry Evans and his wife, Jane Evans. Henry, who was just forty years old when he suffered a brainstem stroke and was left quadriplegic without the ability to speak, saw a television program on robot technology and realized it held hope for him. The result was Robots for Humanity, a collaboration of Willow Garage, Georgia Tech's Healthcare Robotics Lab, Oregon State University, and the Evans family.

Henry, who can move his head and one thumb, uses a special computer mouse to operate a PR2. In a video, Henry is shown manipulating the robot through his computer to get a towel from a drawer and as the robot held it aloft, Henry is able to dry his own face—the first time he could do so in many years. He can also shave himself for the first time, by having the robot hold the electric razor while Henry moves his face. Henry also told the researchers he'd like to be able to give out trick-or-treat candy to children, an application the researchers would have never considered. "We took the robot to a local mall and had Henry operate the robot to put candy in the bags," said Matei. "One of the important things for Henry is social interaction. He came up with this thing. The kids loved it, but we're not sure how many understood they were getting candy from the man and not just the robot. The kids were lining up behind the robot—little kids waited forty-five minutes to get their candy."

Through their work with Henry, the researchers have learned a lot about the challenges of operating a robot in a home environment, lessons they plan to use for the benefit of older adults wanting to age in place. Safety with a frail person is certainly one challenge. Another is the immense variability in each home. "A robot needs to deal with a very wide range of scenarios, and it's extremely difficult," Matai said. "For example, when the robot was navigating in Henry's house, it has windows with curtains. The robot's fans were causing the curtains to billow out. The robot thought it was trapped by a moving wall of obstacles. It's impossible to predict all of these things that can happen in a human house." In contrast, in a factory the environment is defined, and robots are kept in cages with no human interaction.

I asked how close we were to voice command of robots. Voice command is an area that is well-established, I was told—but not when people speak in a normal conversational way. For example, a robot could understand a straight-forward command to pick up a cup from a table. "But if you said, 'Would you be so kind and get me the red cup with a handle, not the glass one,' it would be lost," Matei said.

So are robots an inevitable part of our future? "I wouldn't call it inevitable," Matei responded. "It's not imposed on us externally. The shortage of careworkers—that's inevitable. The robotic technology helping with that is needed, and I'm looking forward to it happening."

Without significant change in working conditions for home health aides, he may be right. There will likely be a growing need for technology to help older people remain at home safely and with independence. "Robots are coming," Jenay believes. "This technology is going to be developed." From her standpoint as a psychologist, the focus needs to be on what older people want from a robot, or it will never be accepted. "It's not what robots *could* do—it's what they *should* do," she said.

But do we really want movable plastic and metal, rather than a warm human, to be our home helpers? The researchers developing tomorrow's robots insist they are meant to help, not replace, human caregivers. But if robots were less expensive, who is to say what the future would be?

In a provocative essay in the journal *Ethics & Medicine*, Jacob Shatzer notes that by posing the choice as "a robot or a nursing home" the argument is over before it begins (in other words, the robot wins, hands down).

> Pushing further, the problem viewed from the perspective of society as a whole seems to be that there are just too many ill and old people. The view of human flourishing, then, is one in which the ill and elderly can be cared for (a noble goal) and continue to live independently. However, the robot solution also seems to propose that for the rest of society flourishing means not having to make the sacrifices necessary to provide care personally or to pay a higher price for the aged to be cared for with dignity by another human being. Finally, success in this model is a mix of noble goals and often ignoble motives: care for the elderly and the chronically ill but in a way that is as inexpensive (in the sense of both financial and emotional investment) as possible.[6]

The Home of the Future

Robots are the most exotic type of home technology being developed for older people or those with disabilities. Far simpler systems are already on the market, from elder-friendly computers to home video monitoring systems, special sensors, and medical devices such as pill dispensers.

Many of these are being tested by older adults and researchers at the Aware Home at Georgia Tech. Computer scientist Brian Jones, manager of the Aware Home Research Initiative, works with a multidisciplinary team of faculty and students to study systems that can let you know you left the refrigerator door ajar or the iron on, confirm that you're picking up the correct pill bottle, remind you you've already fed the cat, and alert health care providers to changes in your blood sugar or sleeping patterns. The idea is to equip our homes with tools that will keep us healthy, connected, entertained, and safe, and even save us money by not wasting energy. While many of the devices are already on the market, the Aware Home Research Initiative is working to integrate and simplify a variety of applications. Study participants come to the Aware Home to try different technologies, and researchers also go to the homes of participants to try devices. Some 370 people have enrolled in the study moving toward its goal of 550.

Older adults with congestive heart failure, one of the most common chronic conditions, can be monitored at a distance to tell how much they've been eating or drinking, how often they got up in the night to go to the bathroom, if they were sleeping in a chair because of breathing discomfort, and so on. While this may sound intrusive, it could be the thing that enables someone to remain in her own home. "Our next step is to develop a baseline of congestive heart failure patients, say, to see if these interventions help them," Brian said.

Will older adults want their homes to be all that "smart"? Do they want to be monitored constantly, even if it's for their own good? According to a study by AARP, eight in ten people sixty-five and older say they would be willing to give up some privacy in order to stay safely in their own homes, and nine in ten said they would be willing to pay for such services.[7]

Technology already exists that people would be willing to use if it were affordable, according to the study. For example, respondents in a survey were interested in devices that would turn off the stove when not in use, regulate the home temperature, or alert family members if daily activity changed (such as not getting out of bed).

Some case studies using telehealth for people with chronic conditions show promise. Partners HealthCare, a Boston-based health system, uses telehealth to help its CHF patients maintain independence and self-manage their disease. Every day patients electronically transmit their weight, blood pressure, pulse, and heart rate to their health care provider. Their care is monitored and coordinated by a nurse, who also conducts patient education and coaching. Twelve hundred patients have participated in the program and overall they have experienced a 50 percent reduction in heart-failure-related hospital admissions. Moreover, the patients were enthusiastic in satisfaction surveys, with 85 percent reporting they felt in control of their health and 82 percent saying they had been able to stay out of the emergency room and the hospital because of the program.[8]

Computers are another obvious tool that can be used to connect older people with friends, family, and professional caregivers; to entertain; and to learn. New ways to simplify computers for those who have never operated one or who have cognitive decline are rapidly advancing through the use of touch screen, video chats, and other applications.

Today's ninety-year-olds have experienced remarkable change in their lifetimes. They grew up when Model A Fords were hot, Charles Lindberg was flying solo for the first time across the Atlantic, and television was a novel invention. But for some, computers and cell phones are way too much technology, let alone robots and fancy sensors and monitoring systems. There is no question, though, that we are rapidly approaching the end of the non-wired generation. Roughly one-third of today's elders over age seventy-five regularly use the Internet for such activities as seeking health information, social networking, or sharing videos, and 77 percent of baby boomers aged fifty to sixty-four are online and half of them are involved in social networking, according to a 2012 Pew Research survey.[9]

A market overview of technology that supports aging in place found four main categories of products:

- Communication and engagement (email, cell and smart phones, videos, games)
- Home safety and security (lifeline alerts, webcams, fall and activity detection)
- Health and wellness (telemedicine, medication management, fitness)
- Learning and contribution (online education, volunteering, working from home)[10]

The report notes many barriers to be overcome before much of the available technology will really catch on including cost; an inability of various electronic gadgets to communicate with each other, either within the home or between ones owned by the older person and others owned by family members (a problem the Aware Home researchers are working on); and a lack of technical support for customers. Of these technologies aimed at helping people age in place, the report found, "The marketplace of products today is fragmented into a cottage industry comprised largely of startups, challenged by both lack of awareness and a difficult economy. But with its fragments assembled into an overall puzzle, this business for boomers and beyond represents a conservative $2 billion market today." By 2020, that figure is projected to be $20 billion.

Without an investment in training not only the elders themselves but also formal and informal caregivers, though, many of the new gadgets may gather dust. Even something like a medication dispenser can be challenging for people with cognitive loss, vision impairment, or other conditions.

Medication dispensers have grown increasingly sophisticated with various locks, lights, and sounds, aimed at both alerting the elder when it's time to take a pill and ensuring that the proper pills are taken. This is actually no small thing. More than one third of people sixty and older take five or more medications; moreover, medication problems contribute to 28 percent of hospital admissions for older adults, according to one study.[11]

In theory, those selling the home-health devices are the ones who train patients to use them. But that training is often poorly done.

Researchers at Georgia Tech interviewed nurses and home health aides about the difficulties of training older people to manage their medications and other tasks. Among the many challenges: literally tens of thousands of medications on the market that have specific doses, side effects, and instructions such as to be taken with or without food; different doctors prescribing medications to one patient without knowing what the patient is already on and different pharmacies dispensing those medications; poor vision on the part of the older person making it difficult to read labels, or arthritic hands that make opening a pill bottle challenging; cognitive decline or a lack of understanding about why it's important to take the prescribed medicines, with many people not taking them if they're feeling okay; and so on. On top of these considerations, dozens of medication dispensing devices are on the market, with no uniformity, and paid caregivers must learn to use different types before training their patients. In addition, many medical tasks that people living at home must perform are more complicated than taking a pill, such as monitoring glucose or using a feeding pump.[12]

Gizmos are also being created that make you wonder. In 2009, researchers at University of Ulster began a project to merge textiles with digital technology. According to a University press release, "The three-year project could have wide-ranging benefits for older people, with electronic devices built in to clothing that could provide information ranging from heart rate and body temperature, to keeping the individual informed of the bus timetable."[13]

At Massachusetts Institute of Technology's Age Lab, researchers were working on a "smart trash can" that would sense when pill bottles were thrown away, as a way to track medication usage, or how much food was tossed, to monitor an elder's sustenance.

Not everyone is thrilled with the push toward technology. British sociology researcher Maggie Mort of Lancaster University has studied telecare being used with older people. Much of the research she reviewed was industry-published and uncritical. When she interviewed older people, she found that many never used the systems that had been installed, saying they were "too complicated, poorly functioning or simply not wanted," she said in an interview published online.[14] Many times people accepted products such as alarm pendants merely to placate family members. They might only use them while doing something risky like climbing a ladder. Others used them to contact the call center just to have a chat because they were lonely. "We thought this was actually rather ingenious. They didn't want to bother relatives or carers but to chat. But, 'just' having a chat is not what the systems are designed to provide. Such behaviour is even termed *misuse* by some service providers."

Other suggestions elders had for improving or adapting telecare systems were generally ignored, she found, with no opportunities for their input. Mort contrasted telecare with simple strategies that elders came up with on their own. For example, one woman had jotted down:

> Arrange things to give peace of mind
> Tel. [telephone] in every room
> Key holders
> My friend and I ring each other every morning
> Neighbours know I am around when my curtains are opened.[15]

In the interview, Mort said, "There is a need for more flexible systems so older people can use them for 'social' reasons, rather than the present care dominated usage."[16] In other words, people were often more interested in using technology as a means to connect and communicate, rather than as a tool for medicalizing their home environment.

Ultimately no matter what technologies are developed, that simple human connection—noticing when your neighbor's curtain is open, a daily call to a friend—may still be what is most important, no matter how sophisticated the technology to come.

CHAPTER 16

What If?

Mapping Our Plan B

Proponents of the alternative models in this book hope that by providing people with that simple human connection, they will be able to avoid, or at least delay, institutional care as they grow old. But it's too soon to tell. Some communities are beginning to struggle with what to do when one of their own gets Alzheimer's, for example—certainly one of the toughest challenges.

Even with the progress people are making to be more intentional about their Third Age, the persistence of denial seems as deeply rooted as an ancient oak. Too often, as I interviewed people, when I asked the difficult question, "What if?" the answer was far from reassuring. I was told, in a vague sort of way, if a member of their community or household became frail or had dementia, she would have to move, usually to an unspecified assisted living facility (the dreaded nursing home was rarely mentioned).

But I was hoping for more. Are there ways that we can still hold close our friends, neighbors, and relatives who can no longer manage in their own homes? Is aging in place (or in community) still just a way station rather than a final destination for many people?

"A lot of times what happens is that these groups start and folks don't realize what they've set themselves up for," reflected Katie McDonough, director of Capitol Hill Village. "They go into it really determined to do what they say they're going to do [help people age in place], but sometimes I wonder if Villages, even Capitol Hill Village at its inception, if they really know what it takes to actually, honestly live out that mission." (In fact, I heard one Village director say she thought *more* of her members should move to assisted living.)

Some organizations have gone the route of referring members to agencies that provide services such as care coordination. The Community Without Walls (see Chapter 7), when it became clear that some of its members needed more support, helped establish a spinoff, Secure@Home, in partnership with a local social service nonprofit. NORCs, such as Penn South and Greenbelt, have a raft of services to extend the time people can remain in their own homes, including care coordination and some home health services. Still, as Nat Yalowitz noted, every year Penn South loses some of its members who move to assisted living or a nursing home.

A few transformative solutions hold the promise that nearly all of us might be able to remain in our own communities. What may be most surprising is that some of these solutions cost far less than the options of assisted living, nursing homes, or full-time paid home care. They require an investment of time, energy, and planning—in short, the sort of forethought that allows us to break through our mass delusion of "It won't happen to me."

Radical Community

Although many cohousing communities would not be able to pull this off, Songaia, near Seattle, provided extraordinary support to a founding member, support that allowed him to remain at home until the end.

When Fred was diagnosed with "Lou Gehrig's" disease (Amyotrophic lateral sclerosis or ALS), he called a community circle to let everyone know. "Then he did something that was quite remarkable," Oz Ragland recalled. "He invited anyone who chose to, to be part of his final journey. He didn't say what that would be like. He said, 'some will say I don't want to watch you die, and some will see it as a rich learning opportunity.'"

The response from many community members was equally remarkable. As he became incapacitated, unable to move his body from the neck down, some of his cohousing friends were willing to provide personal care. "So we were feeding him at our common meals and helping transfer him with a Hoyer lift," Oz said.

Nine months before Fred died, the family hired a part-time caregiver because it had gotten to be more than informal caregivers could manage. With Fred's hospice benefit, the care was affordable.

The children of the community were also very much involved in Fred's care. Eleven-year-old Ian rubbed Fred's feet every night, to help with loss of circulation.

"There's these relationships that are very deep," said Oz.

Another kid, Lucas, came over and took dictation. Fred was working on a book, and Lucas was typing and interacting to get the words down on the computer. Other people would hang out and talk with Fred. Different people were able to bring different things to the relationship.

I was one of the relatively few who could talk comfortably about death. The night that he passed, several of us in the community sang to him. Then there was a family thing at the end. They were all present when he passed. Some were on Skype. He had kids in Scotland and Finland. All the rest of us felt very much a part of it. We saw that everyone who was part of it is much more comfortable with the idea of dying. We saw a good death that had horrible physical aspects to it, but we saw this man with an indomitable spirit.

Oz had shot video clips of Fred thanking each member of the community. After he died, Oz sat individually with each resident and shared Fred's video. "A number were in tears," he said. "An older woman said 'I didn't know he felt like that about me.' She had given Fred two massages a week."

What was amazing, said Oz, was that Fred never asked for help or in any way made people feel guilty if they were uncomfortable facing his dying process. "He invited us to participate," he said. "That's really different. They brought an ethic, he and the other founders, to who we are. We were clear to be a community and enjoy life and to care for each other."

According to Oz, as of late 2012, not a single person had had to move to assisted living or a nursing home from Songaia in its twenty-two years. "Our oldest member broke her hip," he said. "She's eighty. She was in a hospital then rehab. We made plans to modify her house. That's the power of community—we immediately started work on creating a space for her to sleep downstairs, created a path she could navigate, because her house was not accessible—we didn't understand in the 1990s that we would need that. It's awfully easy to ignore."

As related in Chapter 4, Fred's example, though rare, is not unique. Jay was able to die peacefully in his Pleasant Hill Cohousing community, surrounded by friends. With a combination of a paid advocate and supportive neighbors and friends, Jay had what we'd all think of as a good death.

Many cohousing communities do not yet have a significant number of "oldest-old" people, so it's too early to say if most could remain in their homes until the end. I asked Oz what cohousing members could realistically expect in the way of support from each other. "It would depend on the extremity and how much care they're able to get," he said. Perhaps more importantly, "It would depend on the relationships they have with the people here. Fred was beloved. Part of my motivation for trying to get some structures in place that are more supportive is that some of us are not so beloved. We would like to have a little more structure in place so that it's more likely we'll get that type of care." For example, the community could accommodate live-in caregivers as needed, either in the common house guestrooms or extra bedrooms in people's homes. "The cohousing communities are very rich in resources of that type," he said.

Full Circle

One of the most revolutionary approaches to aging in community until the end was developed by a family doctor in a small town in Maine. Allan Teel, MD, was frustrated with the quality of life in nursing homes. He was convinced that many, if not most, people he saw who ended up in dreaded institutions did not have to be there, and he witnessed the stubborn refusal of vulnerable elders to leave their long-time homes. In his book, *Alone and Invisible No More: How Grassroots Community Action and 21st Century Technologies Can Empower Elders to Stay in Their Homes and Lead Healthier, Happier Lives*, he wrote, "Most elders can live in an ordinary residential setting or in their own homes quite safely and quite successfully. We need to stop assuming otherwise and start the transformation back to a successful aging model that emphasizes community and human interaction and deemphasizes the institution and government regulation disguised as protection."[1]

Dr. Teel developed several affordable and comfortable assisted living homes in the community, but he still wasn't satisfied. He went on to create a visionary and affordable in-home program that combines available technology with "a circle of caring," made up of family members, neighbors, and volunteers. To spread the model, he has developed a turnkey business, called Full Circle America, that he hopes compassionate entrepreneurs or nonprofit agencies might replicate.

I visited Maine in October 2012 along with Gail Kohn, who was curious if the model would work for Capitol Hill Village. We flew to Manchester, New Hampshire, and drove three hours to the picturesque town of Damariscotta, not far from the coast. The modest headquarters of Full Circle America are in a two-story building, up a steep flight of stairs over a large thrift shop. We met Dr. Teel ("Chip") and his right-hand staffer, Kim Fenn, in a conference room with a long table and a laptop set up to show us a PowerPoint presentation. Stacks of his book and other reports were piled on tables against the wall.

Chip is affable yet clearly consumed by his mission. He believes passionately that elders have hidden, untapped resources, and that those who wish to support them should focus on each elder's strengths and wishes. Concerns about safety must be balanced with maintaining a high quality of life and that means that older people retain the right to take risks. "Elders accept risk readily," he points out. "Our job is to help individuals achieve their goals and aspirations. That might mean they live on the edge because that's where they want to live."

To affordably keep people in their own homes as long as they wish—and far longer than many believe possible—Full Circle uses monitoring technology, including cameras. Essentially, the vulnerable elder gives up some privacy in exchange for being able to remain at home. With the monitoring systems and volunteers, one employee can look out for fifty in-home elders, making the program extremely affordable—$399 a month, in addition to a limited number of hours for paid hands-on caregivers. Chip's clients pay an average of less than $1,000 a month for Full Circle and paid help combined. This contrasts with the national average monthly cost for a nursing home of more than $6,000, or a whopping $8,000 a month in Maine for a *shared room*.[2]

What Chip has discovered—and what will likely not be a surprise to people who have spent time in nursing homes—is that the actual hands-on care in a facility for an individual resident can be pretty limited in any twenty-four-hour period—the national average is less than 1.5 hours of care per day for each resident by nurses, and 2.35 hours by nursing assistants.[3] (It's worth noting that such data is self-reported by nursing homes, based on a two-week period prior to a state survey being conducted.)[4] Thus much of the cost of nursing home care is really for room and board and administration. For people with dementia, who make up nearly half the nursing home population, "nursing" care may not be as necessary as monitoring and medication reminders, which can be done by volunteers or family members. Yet providing in-home round-the-clock monitoring is so time-consuming for families or costly for paid help that many elders wind up in long-term care facilities.

Chip has been able to turn that around, even for those with the greatest needs. "So we have had people with profound physical and mental impairments who we've been able to take care of remarkably well," he said. "The message I'm trying to get out there is that there is hardly any subgroup that cannot be cared for in their own home. You just might have to throw a few more on-site people-resources into that mix.

"For example, a woman who's had dramatic dementia for fifteen years now, who tells you she goes to the mailbox every day and hasn't been out of her house in a decade, she is content listening to music, reading the newspaper, playing solitaire. She mostly dresses herself, she is ambulatory enough to know when she has to pee. She wouldn't eat unless someone put food in front of her. She's really content where she is. Her family had nearly exhausted hers and their financial resources paying for twenty-four-hour care for her.

We've been able to do half-an-hour in the morning, and half-an-hour in the evening, and twenty-three hours of remote monitoring, all built around the fact of her basic day, rather than her MME [a mental competency exam]. Who cares that she doesn't know who the president is? The real issue is how does she cope with her activities of daily living and what makes her happy or not, what kind of social support does she need. If you look at crafting a plan around it, the job isn't that difficult."

Chip's model depends in part on technology. The tools evolve constantly, but essentially include a personal emergency reporting system (PERS) or life-line, at least one webcam monitoring camera, a special Skype telephone, and various sensors as needed, such as one that gauges the room temperature, prompted by a member who nearly froze to death when her furnace went off, and she didn't know to alert someone. All sorts of other gizmos can be installed for a relatively nominal cost, such as blood pressure and blood sugar monitoring systems and prescription drug dispensers.

It all sounded too good to be true, and Gail and I were eager to see Full Circle in operation.

We clambered into Kim's car and set off to meet Nancy, Full Circle's "star volunteer" who now needed a hand herself. Her house was small and tidy with a lovely flower garden in the back, like so many homes in the area. She had fallen recently and was using a walker. She had a glowing smile and wore large thick glasses.

"I read about [Full Circle] and thought it was just marvelous," she said, after we settled into her cozy living room. She was happy to sign up to volunteer.

"The first person I volunteered with died soon after. One day he got mad at me because I tried to help too much," she said.

"He didn't know how to accept help," Kim observed, a common problem.

"It's hard for people," Nancy agreed. "We want to be the helper, not the helped. The second person ['Nora'] I had was in constant pain and very discouraged. I've become very fond of her. Now she's totally changed. She's done a turn around. She had ended up on a psychiatric ward. Now she's doing chair yoga and tootles around and she's been very concerned about me. Once a week we go out to lunch, then talk on the phone." Nancy was one of three volunteers who helped Nora.

Kim explained that she and the volunteers plan activities based on what the member wants to do, not on some prescribed calendar of activities. Kim always has plenty in her bag of tricks to entice homebodies. Full Circle tries to get each member, no matter his or her challenges, to commit to getting outside the home for nonmedical activities at least once or twice a month. Such experiences might mean going out to lunch at a restaurant, church, or senior center; joining a supper club; seeing a movie, taking a class, or attending a lecture; cooking a meal or doing a home repair for someone else; offering companionship to another member; or teaching a young person to bake or sew.

"I love it," Nancy said of the program. "And look at what it's done for me." She gave a nod to Kim, who had been quietly setting up a new lifeline emergency call system for Nancy as we've talked.

"You know you have a lot of people who would drop everything and come to you," Kim told her.

We headed back out to go to Rockland. It was a cool foggy day with a misty rain, making the small towns look as muted and lovely as an Impressionist painting. Flowers grew in profusion, and when we reached Rockland, the harbor was filled with sailboats.

Our next stop was the home of Nora's sister, "Adele." Adele had found herself in an awkward position when Nora wanted to move in with her. Adele had lost her husband, who had multiple sclerosis, after being his caregiver for many years. Nora too was a widow, and she suffered with chronic pain and mental illness—more than Adele felt she could handle. Adele suggested Nora move to a retirement community, but she was not accepted because of her conditions.

"That freaked us both out," Adele said. "She lives quite close by. She didn't have a social network. I tried to get her involved in a church or social group. It was really hard for her. Then I heard about Full Circle—Nora was resistant to that at first too." Her sister didn't like the lifeline monitor, and she didn't like having to pay a monthly fee.

"Kim started meeting with her," Adele continued. "Then she met Patty [another member] who liked the opera. [Nora] began to meet people. Helpers came in, two at first. Then Kim." Adele had requested three visits a week. "She has accepted that help. She sees the volunteers as friends. She had a woman who was older, then a young helper. I feel that it has created a circle of friends. And it's the first time in her life she's had that. Now she's an advocate for Full Circle. That's new—her confidence. She has something to talk about besides her pain."

Adele said she convinced her sister to go along with the monitoring by telling her she was helping others by trying it out. "This is new technology," she said. "I feel that is a very important aspect of this—but it's the personal connection that's most important." When Nancy became ill, Adele suggested Nora check in on her, for a change. "She's getting a sense of purpose which she hadn't had," she said.

We next visited Patty, the friend who shares a love of opera with Nora. Also at Patty's home was her daughter Amy. Patty and Amy are quite the mother-daughter team. Patty is a strawberry blond, very fit and well put-together, with a beaming smile and severe dementia and aphasia. She lives alone in a roomy townhouse, with Amy living not far away. Amy is a kindergarten teacher and devoted caregiver to her mom. They obviously adore each other.

They both greeted us with warm hugs, as if we were long-lost friends. The kitchen was inviting, with beautiful baskets hanging from the ceiling, many of them made by Patty. She also hooks rugs and makes other crafts—or at least she did in the past. They showed us a note written with a marker on a white board, left by Kaitlin, a helper, letting Amy know how Patty had spent her morning. Patty and Kaitlin had gone on a walk around the picturesque harbor, a favorite spot of Patty's. The white board is one of Full Circle's many simple low-cost solutions for communicating among the various players in a given elder's life. The elder herself, if she's going out for lunch and doesn't want anyone to worry, can jot down that she'll be out. The webcam can pan to the board so Full Circle's human monitors can view it from their computers.

Amy respectfully asked her mother if it would be all right if Amy explained to us Patty's situation. Patty agreed. It was clear that she would not be able to hold her own in a conversation, although she seemed very attentive.

"We saw Dr. Teel on the local news," Amy began. "We thought that [Full Circle] sounds interesting."

Patty responded to everything Amy said with a testimonial, yes, yes, that's right, that's right, nodding her head vigorously.

"Mom had just moved here," Amy went on. "She didn't know anybody. One of the biggest things with Full Circle is all of a sudden you've got new friends, you've got a family—family with a purpose. It's also recognizing Mom saying, 'I want to stay with my things, in my own house.'"

"Bor-ing," Patty interjected. I took it to mean that it was boring when she first came and had no friends.

"We needed more," Amy said. "We looked at assisted living and nursing homes. What you get there is a bedroom. You're locked into a rigorous schedule. It's more like day care for elders, rather than allowing people to have power over their lives." With the words "nursing home," Patty looked concerned and said, "No, no."

Amy contacted Full Circle and met Kim at a bakery. "We talked and got a feel for each other," she said. "We met three or four times and decided this is exactly what we needed. It started with the technology but you need more than technology—"

"That's nothing," Patty put in.

"You need the people," Amy said.

"That's it!" Patty said happily. "That's us."

Amy looked at her mother and said with portent, "The opera."

"Oh, the opera!" Patty said. She turned to Kim and asked, "Are we going? It's wonderful! I cry!"

Kim had organized a group of Full Circle members and volunteers to go to see a local high-definition streaming of the Metropolitan Opera.

Amy said, "It was an immediate connection."

"That was a big one," Patty agreed.

With Full Circle, Amy had a way to find friends for Patty. The volunteers range from twenty-two to eighty-something years old. They'll pick up prescriptions or run other errands for Patty, or just spend time with her.

Amy then asked Patty to show me a special phone that allowed Patty to easily Skype directly through the phone, instead of on a computer, part of Full Circle's technology. On a touch screen were photos of Amy and Kim and others whom Patty could call simply by touching the photo. Usually, though, others initiate calls to Patty, said Amy, implying that even that simple task would be difficult for her mother.

Patty's other daughter lives in Texas and is a foster mother. She can show Patty the babies she cares for through the Skype camera. They told us about a time when Patty was at Amy's house. Through the webcam they could view Patty's beloved cat, wandering about her house, which delighted Patty.

Kim pointed out the webcam, a small white device that pans across Patty's downstairs and shows the image through the Internet. Amy explained there is a monitoring camera upstairs as well. Full Circle's paid monitors can view real-time images when they check on clients, which can be several times a day, depending on the elder's need.

"I don't get that," Patty said of the webcam.

Amy tried to explain it to her. Patty laughed when I assured her, "I don't get it either."

"It gives me peace of mind," Amy said. "I could hire some techie person and put similar equipment in my mom's home. But who would monitor it? It's not something you'd do by yourself."

"No, no, that's not the thing," Patty offered.

Patty asked us if we'd walked by the harbor. When I said we hadn't had a chance, she said, "Oh goodness. Go! Go! It's beautiful."

Kim spoke up and said the program allows them to adapt regularly to suit Patty's changing needs. "It's different every week," she said. "Sometimes we take you to cheer up someone else," she said to Patty, letting her know she's making her own contribution.

Patty is not safe to walk alone anymore, and she no longer drives. But, Amy said, she likes fixing her own breakfast.

After a delightful visit, we head back to the car. Kim gave us a reality check of the serene picture Patty presented. Sitting at her computer at ten o'clock one night, Kim decided to do one last monitoring check of Patty. On her screen, she could see Patty walking around her house with a candle and a fire starter. Kim immediately called Amy who rushed over to the house. Patty became angry with her daughter. Kim attributed Patty's agitation to a form of "sundowner's syndrome"—a common condition associated with Alzheimer's disease when people experience bouts of anger, restlessness, and fear.

As part of Full Circle's philosophy, Kim was trying to come up with ways that Patty could make a contribution and give her life more meaning. One idea was to team her up with a Meals on Wheels volunteer. Patty, very fit and friendly, could be the one who takes the meal from the car to the recipient's door.

As we're in the car, Kim shared some of her own background. She began with Full Circle working on the company's website and promotion but soon morphed into a jill-of-all-trades, part social worker, friend, administrator, home monitor, and on and on. She seemed to share Chip's passion for their mission. She told of visiting a nursing home where a resident approached her. "He took my hand and said, 'This is the loneliest place I've ever been,'" she said. That incident was one reason she was so motivated to honor members' wishes to remain in their own homes, supported by people like her and Full Circle volunteers.

The following day, Chip took us to visit Marty, ninety-two. He lived in a large house at the edge of the woods that he and his late wife had had built. We entered into a spacious room with a cathedral ceiling and magnificent brick fireplace, fit for Beowulf. Marty was an artist and the house was a jumble of his paintings stacked everywhere. In the middle of the living room was an easel.

He had earned a degree from the Museum of Fine Arts in Boston. He was also a retired Air Force pilot and a long-time church deacon. "I keep busy," he said. "I don't like rocking chairs."

A heavy-set man, a bit unkempt, he now used a walker. His mind and wit were sharp.

During the Depression, he told us, he had worked in a bookbindery for Houghton Mifflin by day and went to school at night. His father had abandoned the family, leaving his mother with three kids, all of whom worked in factories to help out the family. In 1955 he was stationed at Loring Air Force Base, alone, while his wife and children were in Boston. On July fourth a friend invited him to Maine. He fell in love with the place, and he and his wife settled in his current house in 1986. His wife lived in a nearby nursing home for six years before she died.

He had signed up for Full Circle after being in a rehab center for five weeks. "I had incidents of falling for no reason," he said. "The doctor at the ER said we'll find out what's wrong with you. They couldn't find anything. But then they checked for diabetes. That's what it was."

Chip asked him if he had considered moving to the nursing home after his last discharge from the hospital.

"It's a legitimate question about whether I should have returned home or not," Marty said matter-of-factly. "I consider this an experiment—a new way of doing something. When I was approached [about Full Circle], I said, 'Why not?' I'll become more enfeebled from natural causes of age, but now I'm capable of managing my own affairs."

He paused to let us know, in so many words, not to overstay our welcome—he was getting ready to go out to lunch shortly. He goes out two or three times a week. I asked if he still drives. With a twinkle in his eye, he responded, "That's a sore subject. The state took my license." He gave Chip a look that suggested he had had a hand in this. "Do I miss driving? Of course. The freedom to come and go when I want." He cooked his own meals and was on a limited diet, he said, because of the diabetes, and he also used Meals on Wheels.

I asked him how he felt about the monitoring technology that Full Circle installed in his home. "It makes me feel secure when they ask where are you," he said. "I think it's a good innovation." (Although he said the monitors spoke to him, Chip said later that was not accurate. For many clients, a disembodied voice would frighten them, so their policy was not to use that feature of the system. At any rate, Marty clearly felt he was being looked after.)

Marty showed us his current work, a series of paintings of Maine lighthouses. "Before my license was taken away, I was doing a series of the Damariscotta River," he said. "The most beautiful parts are the headwaters of Damariscotta Lake—[known as] The Thread of Life." He recently had an exhibit at a local church.

As for Full Circle, he said, "As it's developing, I'm more comfortable with it. The aide who comes and her assistant do beautiful work around here. I'm really a slob. They come twice a week. I have a lady friend who comes on Thursdays. And another friend brings me breakfast every Tuesdays—we have oatmeal and coffee and chew the fat." The previous evening his good friends brought him dinner and hung out for a couple of hours.

I asked him if he gets lonely. "I have times when I could have felt better," he said. "But I paint and the time just flies away. People need whatever their talents or professions are—they need to do it. You can't sit here twenty-four hours a day and not do anything. It won't work. I make it a point to have my friends visit when they want. And I go out. I used to give my friend Al communion when he had medical problems, and now Al comes to visit me."

"Letting other people do things for you is giving them opportunities to feel good," Chip noted.

Marty agreed. "People want to help, but they don't want to invade your privacy," he said. "I let it be known whenever you want to wash the floor—have at it! It's the little things that matter. Whether taking the trash or washing the floor. I guess I could do it myself, but I'm too damn lazy. Almost daily I get calls from people offering to stop by the store for me. Another part of the reality, I must admit, I deliberately want people to come, and I let them know it. I know what the alternative is—sitting here alone would probably kill me."

The transportation issue was a serious problem, he added. Every Saturday evening two friends take him to mass and bring him home, for which he is grateful.

We said our good-byes so that he could get ready for his lunch date. I admired his candor, his humor, and his willingness to accept help.

Later Chip picked up on Marty's comments about transportation. It is indeed a big issue for people who can no longer drive. Providing free or paid transport to frail elders as often as they might want or need it is a Sisyphean task, Chip believes. He points to his own father, who is frail and incontinent. For someone to pick him up to go somewhere, "It might take two hours on both ends, by the time you help him get dressed, then it's time for him to go to the bathroom, and so on. So paying for transportation to adult day care is not sustainable," he said.

With the technology and supportive network, he said, you can achieve some of the goals of getting out though. "Take going to church," he said. "Maybe they could go once a month, and then videostream the other Sundays. There's a blend you have to have of streaming and transporting.

"Then there's the people part—you need to engage the elders themselves, you need to engage the families," he said. "Right now the families are overwhelmed." His vision is along the lines of "it takes a village." People who encounter the homebound elder—perhaps the cleaning lady, newspaper delivery person, letter carrier, or lawn-care service—need to be enlisted to help be the eyes, ears, and friendly voice to ask how the person is getting along. For example, a woman in his father's neighborhood has a small convenience store and restaurant. She delivers prepared meals to a few people as a business.

When she delivers food to her father, they've arranged for her to give him his evening pills.

How many people have the kind of networks in their community to put all this together is not clear. In a small town like Damariscotta it may be easier than say, Los Angeles. Still, the main point is to be creative, to look beyond the usual social service agency and nuclear family models to enlist others who may be quite willing to help in small, specific ways.

"How do we use limited human resources to accomplish this?" Kim said. "We have to act as a catalyst more than a volunteer coordinator. [The elders] then build connections themselves." She noted that Patty, who is seventy-seven, helps Nora, also seventy-seven, in and out of the car, because Patty perceives Nora as worse off than she is. The point is to draw on the generosity and abilities of Full Circle members themselves, much as the Village model tries to do.

Chip and Kim's next challenge seems tougher than creating Full Circle: spreading the model across the nation. Chip is frustrated by the slow pace of progress and the lack of support from federal and state funding agencies, which he argues would save hundreds of millions of dollars through his approach. With his own resources—including his retirement savings and home equity—and some foundation grants, he had mustered a marketing campaign that he described as "slow and rinky-dink."

"I really believe there are grassroots groups ready and willing, but the amount of handholding is huge," he said. "In medicalizing this model, everybody is terrified they're going to screw up." Still, he's making progress. In early 2013 he was collaborating on a dozen grassroots initiatives in seven states.

One was Capitol Hill Village. Gail Kohn had returned to Maine with CHV director Katie McDonough and Robert Jenkens, senior vice president of the National Cooperative Bank.

I was curious what Robert Jenkens, who has worked to transform aging services for many years, thought about Full Circle. "Chip has figured out a way to take technology, the benefits of the monitoring, and then very effectively combine it with the hands-on formal and informal capacity," Robert Jenkens told me. "It's the integration that makes it powerful."

Chip has also broken down two taboos, Jenkens said. One was the assumption that people would never allow monitoring cameras in their homes; the other was that in-home care was too expensive for most people. By relying on a team of informal volunteers and family members, Full Circle has demonstrated an affordable way to provide care, even to people with serious and unpredictable conditions and of modest means.

It also showed that older people would accept monitoring as a reasonable trade-off for staying in their homes.

Jenkens considers Full Circle a model that is "very replicable," with its turnkey business template. "There's a very clear structure which is articulated, and there's a profit motive," he said. "Once you create a profit motive and a structure, you should be able to replicate it."

Gail Kohn thought that Capitol Hill Village was an ideal grassroots organization to act as a "beta testing" site for Full Circle. Each year, Gail said, CHV loses about five members who must go to assisted living or a nursing home. CHV and a few other Villages in Washington are moving forward with a pilot project, to learn if Full Circle can help their most frail members remain in their homes.

House Calls and Green Houses

Full Circle is not the only avenue being pursued by Capitol Hill Village to help its most vulnerable members stay in the community. From its inception, CHV had the long view of what it means to put in place the services their members would need if they became homebound. "What Gail did that's different than a lot of Villages, she didn't ignore that problem," said Katie McDonough. "She didn't ignore issues that families were coming to her with. A lot of Villages ignore them or they say we can't handle that, or they push it off to a fee-for-service organization. What we embrace here—if we're going to be honest about the mission, we have to face these challenges, even if it's taxing on the organization. We have to push ourselves to figure out a way to respond to people."

At first, they hired a social worker (Katie McDonough, before being promoted to executive director) to handle care coordination for those most in need, or they steered members to a private-pay geriatric care manager. But that was not sustainable. More staff would be needed to provide care management in-house, and hiring professionals "is not true to our mission," said Katie. "What we're doing here is about a community of people helping each other address these challenges."

The organization is now launching a program using specially-trained volunteers to each be the point-person for a frail member at risk of having to move to an institutional setting. One volunteer is matched with one homebound elder. Depending on the individual's needs, the volunteer may check in by phone every day, visit once a week, or some combination of calls and visits.

The volunteers, then, are the eyes and ears, who then will alert CHV staff about problems that arise. This will allow the social worker to be more "out in front" of people, to try to prevent falls or catch a stroke and get the person to a doctor, before a crisis occurs. The volunteers will also help keep the elders plugged in. "These people isolate themselves as they get more frail," Katie said. "They don't go out as much, they don't self-advocate as much. The way we've been operating, we tell people you can call us and tell us what you need. But not everybody's doing that. If you have had changes in your cognition or you're not feeling well, you might not be able to call. We want to make sure we're still engaging those people."

In addition to the care coordination, CHV partnered with a local Medical House Calls program to bring physicians and nurse practitioners to the homes of those who have difficulty getting to the doctor. "If it weren't for Medical House Calls we'd have members who would not be at home or would have died by now because they'd want to stay at home. The Medical House Calls program is bringing vital primary care services to people on a regular basis," Katie said.

The doctors work as a team with nurses, pharmacists, social workers, and others in a holistic way. The medical team includes CHV staff members who can share their perspective on how the member is doing.

Even with all these efforts, CHV recognizes that a handful of members may not be able to remain at home. Here too, CHV is creatively finding a way to keep people in their community, if not in their own home. Under Gail's leadership, CHV is partnering with other local nonprofits to develop a small-house model to deliver noninstitutional nursing-home-level care in neighborhoods throughout Washington.

Known as Green Houses, the small-house model is the brainchild of Dr. Bill Thomas, who made a name in the world of long-term care by breaking the mold of the nursing home. After years of trying to reform nursing homes from within through an approach he dubbed the Eden Alternative, Bill Thomas became convinced it was an impossible task; the only way to get rid of institutional care and poor quality of life, he believes, is by starting from scratch. The result is the Green House, which looks like a normal large single-story home.

A dozen or so elders live there, with each person having his or her own bedroom and bath. The spacious open country kitchen, living room, dining room, and outdoor space are shared. Specially-trained staff called *shahbazim* (meaning royal falcons in Persian) combine the roles of nurse's aide, homemaker, and companion. Other services—nursing, physical therapy, physician—are brought to the home. The model is widely admired and has been found to deliver high levels of resident and family satisfaction and medical care.

Until recently Green Houses had been built only on the campuses of retirement communities. But now innovators are planting them in residential neighborhoods. The first to do so was St. John's in Rochester, New York, in 2011, and another was built in Baltimore by a nonprofit faith-based development corporation in 2012. I visited both with Gail Kohn, as part of our mutual interest in learning just how far "aging in community" can be extended.

In Rochester two Green Houses were built side-by-side to blend into the surroundings of a suburban housing development. We spent an hour or so at one of the homes, where we saw a glimpse of daily life. The *shahbazim* were preparing lunch and playing cards with the elders. We were told that families come a lot more often to visit, compared to when their loved ones lived in the large nursing home on St. John's campus. Family members have their own house keys and are welcome to stay for a meal at no charge. Everyone eats around the long dining room table, part of Bill Thomas's philosophy of *convivium*. People also share old family recipes, we were told, such as one man, Sal, whose family spaghetti sauce had been prepared and served. The *shahbazim* prepare the food, with help from elders if they wish, so the enticing aromas of home cooking are part of everyday life, unlike a nursing home where a central kitchen cooks mass quantities of food that are often delivered on trays.

The Green Houses in Rochester were unusually spacious, as were the private bedrooms, each with a double bed and personal belongings decorating the space. The backyard was filled with birdfeeders and raised garden beds allowing elders to plant vegetables and flowers.

Dorothy, who had moved there from the original St. John's nursing home, said she loves having a private room. When she lived in "the big house," her roommate was "senile," she said, and that was difficult. People could get outside in the traditional nursing home, but only at prescribed times, and then, "They'd make you go back inside." Here, people could go outside whenever they wish.

Mimi, the recreational therapist, sees her role as supporting the *shahbazim* as they do "natural things" with the elders. Instead of bingo every Tuesday, days unfold organically: lingering over the dining room table with a second cup of coffee and the newspaper, playing cards, setting the table, helping bake, puttering in the garden.

The staff was pleased to report that neighbors were welcoming, and in fact a couple of them had even expressed interest in getting on a waiting list to reserve a spot in the Green House if they needed it someday—hardly a typical request for a nursing home.

Another new Green House community was built on the grounds of baseball's old Memorial Stadium in Baltimore. Although not quite as close to neighbors as the Rochester houses, the Green House at Stadium Place seems a good fit for urban Baltimore, with each Green House taking up one story of a new four-story building. They retain the same features of other Green Houses with one bonus: each floor overlooks the playing field of Cal Ripken Youth Development Park, where at-risk youth come to play ball. The elders can sit on the wide screened porch, drinking lemonade or Pabst Blue Ribbon, watching the kids shag fly balls, or they can go down closer to the action behind home plate.

As pleasant as the Rochester and Baltimore Green Houses are, the residents do not necessarily come from the immediate neighborhood. What Gail Kohn envisions for Capitol Hill is different.

Along with other nonprofits with expertise in long-term care and affordable housing, Capitol Hill Village is working on a project that will bring Green Houses to several Washington, DC, neighborhoods. One will be built in the Capitol Hill neighborhood, with the idea that CHV members no longer able to stay in their own homes will be able to stay in the community, connected to long-time friends, neighbors, and familiar surroundings. With a comprehensive set of options in place—the social and transportation support of other Village members, volunteer care coordinators, Full Circle technology, Medical House Calls, the Green House—Capitol Hill Village envisions a future where all its members can truly age in community.

Katie McDonough said it can be frustrating that there is not better support for addressing long-term care challenges. Aging in place and long-term care, she said,

> is something as a larger society we need to address together. But because we're not addressing it, it's devolving to communities and individuals, and we're not really getting any help from anyone. We're doing it on a shoestring budget, and we're trying to figure out how to do it in a way that is efficient and locally based. What we're doing is right, but how to make it financially stable in the long term is the question that we have to continually ask ourselves, and nobody really has the answer yet.

She's convinced, though, that their small-scale approach, rooted in relationships, is the path forward. "It's like we're a little wheel trying to direct this huge Mack truck," she said of their efforts to transform the system. "We want to say, 'We're important, you need to pay attention!'"

Home- and Community-Based Services

In addition to these independent efforts, federal and state governments are experimenting with ways to bring home- and community-based services to vulnerable elders to prevent institutionalization. PACE—Program of All-Inclusive Care for the Elderly—has its roots in the Chinatown–North Beach section of San Francisco, where, in the 1970s, a visionary public health dentist, William Gee, along with a handful of other community leaders, sought a new way to serve the needs of immigrant elders. The basic idea is to bring a full raft of services to older people in their homes and in neighborhood adult day centers, allowing people who are eligible for nursing home level care to remain at home. Most have incomes that make them eligible for Medicaid. The program is "capitated," meaning each person receives all services, including nursing home if it comes to that, for a set annual fee. It is thus in the program's interest to keep participants as healthy as possible.

As of 2012, there were ninety-two PACE programs and two Pre-PACE programs operating in thirty-one states.[5] The average PACE participant is eighty years old with a staggering "7.9 medical conditions" and in need of assistance with three activities of daily living, such as bathing or dressing. Nearly half have dementia. Yet almost all—90 percent—still live in their own homes.

PACE participants come to a central location a few times during the week as needed for hot meals, companionship, physical therapy, and coordination of all their services. A van provides transportation, and all services are covered, even eyeglasses, dentures, and hearing aids, unlike traditional Medicare. While the program is somewhat less costly than a nursing home, its main benefit is keeping people healthy enough to live in their own homes and communities, where they wish to be. By coming frequently to an adult day center, elders also find more companionship than if they were isolated in their homes. As one participant at Hopkins Elder Plus, a PACE program in Baltimore, put it, "They told me it was like family. I didn't feel that way at first, but now I do."

Another new approach, called structured family caregiving, is being piloted in Ohio, Indiana, Rhode Island, and Massachusetts. In this model, a family member is paid a stipend to care for their loved one, backed by a clinical team that includes a nurse and a social worker. According to an article in

Healthcare Finance News, states are saving millions in Medicaid funds through the program. In Massachusetts, for example, the daily nursing home rate is $172. In comparison the state's structured family program, called SeniorLink, receives $83 a day per client. Of this, 60 percent goes to the family caregiver and the balance pays for the clinical team and administration. Massachusetts saved $130–$140 million in 2012 through the program. Although the family stipend amounts to just $17,000 a year, most participants are low-income people who are not earning much more than that in the workforce, the article noted.[6]

Although all these efforts seem Lilliputian when contrasted with the nursing home behemoth, the trend is promising.

"Where I have seen success and innovations with outcomes and sustainability is where we break down the scale and base the solution on human relationships," said Robert Jenkens. "I think that's a pretty good guide for anything we're looking at—does it break down the scale so true relationships can form. If it doesn't get to the scale and the relationships and the flexibility that's implied with that, so the services support the person's preferences, the solutions will not be good. If we can do that, whether it's person-directed care, Green Houses, or Villages, then we'll have seen a sea change."

Epilogue

As I was completing the manuscript of this book, our neighbor Ann sent an email inviting those of us on our block who are sixty and older to a potluck. She and her husband Merrill wanted to discuss aging in place here in our neighborhood. "I realize that for now, everyone's mostly healthy and independent, so there might not be too much interest just yet," she wrote. "But if there is, we'd like to discuss what, if anything, folks have thought about becoming aged, staying in our homes, and building some kind of cooperative network among us."

We have a close-knit neighborhood, but still, Ann was surprised when twenty-two people from a three-block area crowded into their living room. Over plates of baked ziti, chicken, and salad, we began a discussion that echoed the themes in the pages of this book. All but one couple, who plan to move to a continuing care retirement community when they reach their early seventies, want to remain on the street. The questions flowed: How would we make our homes accessible? How would we ensure people felt comfortable asking for help? What kinds of help were reasonable to expect? Should we include the younger families in our network?

By the end of the gathering, we were launched. I realized how far ahead of the curve we were. We were proactively pushing back against the entrenched denial that we were growing older. More important, we were building our network on a firm foundation of trust. We had all lived in our neighborhood for many decades, helping each other through illness, the death of loved ones, new babies, retirement, bar mitzvahs, and other assorted milestones. We had spent countless picnics and New Year's Eves together. While we are not all close confidantes, we have each other's back.

Even before our second meeting, one creative couple was working on a website for our little group. It has photos from various gatherings, some of them hilarious, as our street is locally famous for lampooning topical issues when we march in our town's July fourth parade. There are links to financial resources like information about reverse mortgages, to adult education courses, and to upcoming events.

We already are dealing with a serious medical issue as one of our own, who grew up on the street, was recently diagnosed with Stage 4 breast cancer. We seamlessly organized meal support and household help for her overwhelmed husband while she was in the hospital. We get regular emails from him about his wife's condition and unflagging spirits. In one he wrote, "We believe the prayers and happy thoughts and positive energy sent her way are working. We thank you. Love and white light to all of you."

I realized that aging in community doesn't begin when we turn a particular age, be it sixty or eighty. It begins right now, whatever our age, forming relationships, lending a hand, sharing a laugh, knowing you're there for each other. That's the lesson from all who shared their stories in this book. It matters not what form or structure our communities take—or if they have no structure at all; the point is to have a community, a circle of caring, made of family, friends, and neighbors, who will be there for the long haul, as best they can, as we live our final chapter.

Glossary of Alternative Models

affinity group—See **niche retirement community**.

aging in place—Remaining in your own home throughout your life, even if you have physical or cognitive challenges.

cohousing—An intentional community, architecturally designed to include a private apartment or house for each resident or family, with shared common spaces to accommodate group meals and gatherings. Usually governed by consensus. Most units are purchased, but some cohousing communities include rental units.

Community Without Walls, Inc. (CWW)—A network of older people dedicated to creating friendship and social opportunities for members, who pay modest dues. Volunteer-run and organized in chapters known as Houses. To date there is one Community Without Walls, in Princeton, New Jersey.

condominium—Similar to a **housing cooperative**, but with different legal and financial arrangements. Residents own their apartments or town-houses, rather than a share of the whole, and generally do not have as strong a sense of community as co-ops, especially those co-ops that are limited-equity. That said, most **cohousing** communities are set up legally as condominiums.

continuing care retirement community (CCRC)—A retirement community owned and operated by a private or nonprofit corporation that includes all levels of care, from independent living to assisted living to skilled nursing and rehabilitation. Payment options vary, but typically a large initial payment in addition to monthly payments includes care for life.

housing cooperative—A member-owned nonprofit housing community, made up of apartments, townhouses, single-family homes, or mobile homes. Co-op member-owners buy a share in the housing cooperative which gives them full rights to their own apartment or house. Cooperatives are democratically run. Some are called "limited equity" to maintain affordability, and others are "market rate," meaning their prices fluctuate with the market.

naturally occurring retirement community (NORC)—Any neighborhood or locale with a significant portion of older people who have aged in place. Those that have created supportive service programs are called NORC-SSPs, or NORCs for short. NORCs are not membership-based but instead serve all older people in the given area who request help. Supportive services may be paid for by municipal or county governments, housing cooperatives, grants, and modest fees.

niche retirement community—An apartment or housing development created on behalf of a constituency who share a common identity, such as sexual orientation, labor union membership, artistic inclination, or religious faith. A niche community may be built by a developer, an entrepreneur, or a nonprofit organization, and houses or apartments may be offered for rent or for sale. Some are affordable; many are not.

retirement community—Age-restricted community, typically for those fifty-five and older. Usually privately owned and operated, with planned activities, public dining areas, and amenities such as fitness rooms, golf courses, or pools. Also known as active adult communities. (See also **continuing care retirement community**.)

Village model—A neighbors-helping-neighbors membership organization, dedicated to helping people age in place. Assistance is typically provided by a combination of volunteers and paid staff. Members have a central contact point for non-medical assistance, such as transportation and home maintenance, as well as for social connections and activities. Members typically pay dues to cover staff and office expenses in addition to raising money through grants, fund raising appeals, and special events.

Questions to Help Guide Our Choices

Would you like to grow old in your current home?

- Is your home suitable if you had mobility problems? If not, do you have the resources and space to adapt it (e.g., adding a first-floor bedroom and bath or installing a chair lift or elevator)? Have you considered consulting a remodeler who specializes in aging in place, to learn what it would take?
- Are you friends with your neighbors? Could you call on them for help from time to time?
- Would you need a car to live where you are now? If you were unable to drive, is there alternative transportation? How far are you from shops, post office, library, church, doctors? Are there safe places to walk?

    Models to consider: the Village, NORC, Community Without Walls, housesharing

Would you like to live in an intentional community?

- Is having a "built-in" set of friends important? (This may be especially valuable if you are single, shy, or lacking a support network.)
- Do you like the idea of living among like-minded people?
- Are you open to sharing common space (yard, community rooms)?
- Would you prefer less maintenance than a single-family home typically requires?
- Are you willing to spend some time volunteering in the community or going to committee meetings?

    Models to consider: Cohousing, niche community, housing cooperatives, Generations of Hope

Are you concerned about your finances?

- Do you need to reduce your living expenses over the long-term?

    Models to consider: Housesharing, limited-equity cooperatives, a few cohousing communities that include reduced-rent units, Generations of Hope

Would you prefer to live among people your own age as you grow older?

- Do you like the idea of having a group of friends your age to hang out with during the day, potentially travel with, or discuss common concerns associated with aging?
- Does the peace and quiet of not living around children appeal to you—or at least not bother you?

    Models to consider: Senior cohousing, some NORCs, senior housing cooperatives, niche communities

Is living among children important to you?

- Do you enjoy the energy of kids around you?
- Does the idea of volunteering with kids or helping a neighbor with babysitting now and then sound fun?

    Models to consider: Generations of Hope, multi-generational cohousing or cooperatives, the Village, some NORCs, family arrangements

Is being near your extended family (e.g., grown children, grandchildren, siblings) important to you?

    Models to consider: New family arrangements, housesharing

Do you want to shake the dice?

- Do you feel you're in a rut in your current living situation? Do you like the idea of living somewhere you've never lived before during the next stage of life? Are you concerned that moving will mean you won't make new friends?

    Models to consider: Niche community, cohousing, Generations of Hope

Notes

CHAPTER 1

1. William H. Thomas, *What Are Old People For? How Elders Will Save the World* (Acton, MA: VanderWyk and Burnham, 2004), 105.

2. W. Andrew Achenbaum, *Old Age in the New Land: The American Experience since 1790* (Baltimore: Johns Hopkins University Press, 1978), 4.

3. Becca R. Levy, Pil H. Chung, Talya Bedford, and Kristina Navrazhina, "Facebook as a Site for Negative Age Stereotypes," *The Geronotologist,* Feb. 7, 2013, *gerontologist.oxfordjournals.org.*

4. Barbara Joyce Bedney, Robert Bruce Goldberg, and Kate Josephson, "Aging in Place in Naturally Occurring Retirement Communities: Transforming Aging Through Supportive Service Programs," *Journal of Housing for the Elderly* 24, no. 3–4 (2010): 316.

5. Judith Graham, "'Elderly' No More," *The New Old Age* (blog), *New York Times,* April 19, 2012, *newoldage.blogs.nytimes.com.*

6. Edward Schumacher-Matos, "Let Me Live Long, but Don't You Dare Call Me Old," *NPR Ombudsman* (blog), March 12, 2013, *www.npr.org/blogs/ombudsman.*

7. Erik Wemple, "Journos: Never Call Someone 'Elderly,'" Erik Wemple (blog), *Washington Post,* March 12, 2013, *www.washingtonpost.com/blogs/erik-wemple.*

8. The Associated Press, *The Associated Press Stylebook 2013* (New York: Basic Books, 2013), 94.

9. "Sun City: 40 Years of Success," accessed Dec. 17, 2013, *suncitylivingaz.com/vc/sun-city-40-years-of-success.*

10. "Modern Living: Man on the Cover: Del Webb," *Time,* Aug. 3, 1962, 49.

11. TW+A Research, "Insights for Attracting Baby Boomer Retirees," *SeniorStat* 1, no. 1 (May 2009), *www.twaresearch.com/newsletters/05_09newsletter.html.*

12. "2010 Del Webb Baby Boomer Survey," *dwboomersurvey.com/2010_Baby_Boomer_Survey.pdf.*

13. "Retirement Communities in the US: Market Research Report," *IBISWorld Industry Report 62331,* October, 2013, *www.ibisworld.com/industry/default.aspx?indid=1599.*

14. "2010 Del Webb Baby Boomer Survey."

15. MetLife Mature Market Institute, *Housing for the 55+ Market: Trends and Insights on Boomers and Beyond* (New York: MetLife Mature Market Institute, 2009), 9, *www.metlife.com.*

16. George Michaelson, "Maggie Kuhn: Gray Panther on the Prowl," *Parade,* Dec. 18, 1977, 8; Muriel R. Glick, *The Denial of Aging: Perpetual Youth, Eternal Life, and Other Dangerous Fantasies* (Cambridge: Harvard University Press, 2007), 226.

17. Andrew D. Blechman, *Leisureville: Adventures in a World Without Children* (New York: Atlantic Monthly Press, 2008).

18. Lou Carlozo, "Rambling Retirees Trade Homes for Boats, RVs, Sofas," *Reuters,* Oct. 5, 2012, *www.reuters.com.*

19. Nat Yalowitz and Ron Caplain, *Faces and Voices: Growing Older in America: The NORC Experience* (New York, Penn South Social Services, 2005), 5.

20. Paul Hawken, *Blessed Unrest: How the Largest Movement in the World Came into Being and Why No One Saw It Coming* (New York: Viking, 2007), 2.

CHAPTER 2

1. Nat Yalowitz, *Growing Older: At Home—Challenges & Opportunities* (New York: The NORC Supportive Services Center, 2007), 1.

2. Stephen M. Golant, "Aging in Place Solutions for Older Americans: Groupthink Responses Not Always in Their Best Interests," *Public Policy & Aging Report,* Winter 2009, 33.

3. MetLife Mature Market Institute, *Aging in Place 2.0: Rethinking Solutions to the Home Care Challenge* (New York: MetLife Mature Market Institute, 2010), 5, *www.metlife.com.*

4. Bill Thomas, "A Revolution in Life Beyond Adulthood," ChangingAging (blog), Aug. 22, 2012, *changingaging.org/blog/a-revolution-in-life-beyond-adulthood.*

5. Ishani Kar-Purkayastha, "An Epidemic of Loneliness," *The Lancet* 376, no. 9758 (2010): 2114.

6. Rana Sampson, "The Problem of Misuse and Abuse of 911," Center for Problem-Oriented Policing, 2002, *www.popcenter.org/problems/911_abuse.*

7. Andrew V. Wister and Thomas K. Burch, "Attitudes of the Elderly Toward Living Arrangements: Conceptual and Methodological Issues," *The Retirement Community Movement: Contemporary Issues,* ed. Leon A. Pastalan, (Binghamton: The Haworth Press, 1989), 12.

8. Teresa A. Kennan, *Home and Community Preferences of the 45+ Population* (Washington, DC: AARP Research & Strategic Analysis, 2010), *www.aarp.org.*

9. Andrew Steptoe, Aparna Shankar, Panayotes Demakakos, and Jane Wardle, "Social Isolation, Loneliness, and All-Cause Mortality in Older Men and Women," *Proceedings of the National Academy of Sciences* 110, no. 15, (2013): 5799, *www.pnas.org.*

10. "Friends Not Children and Grandchildren Could Be the Key to a Happy Retirement," University of Greenwich, April 21, 2010, *www2.gre.ac.uk.*

11. Neena L. Chappell and Mark Badger, "Social Isolation and Well-Being," *Journal of Gerontology* 44, no. 5 (1989): 169–76.

12. Cari Jo Clark, et al., "Neighborhood Cohesion is Associated with Reduced Risk of Stroke Mortality," *Stroke* (online edition), April 14, 2011, *www.ncbi.nlm.nih. gov/pmc/articles/PMC3102433/.*

13. Lynne C. Giles, Gary F.V. Glonek, Mary A. Luszcz, Gary R. Andrews, "Effects of Social Networks on 10-Year Survival in Very Old Australians: The Australian

Longitudinal Study of Aging," *Journal of Epidemiology & Community Health* 59 (2005): 578.

14. Midlife in the United States (MIDUS), *Subjective Aging: Importance of How Old You Feel* (Madison, WI: Institute on Aging, University of Wisconsin, 2011), *aging.wisc.edu/midus/newsletter/index.php.*

15. Dan Buettner, *The Blue Zones: Lessons for Living Longer from the People Who've Lived the Longest* (Washington, DC: National Geographic Society, 2008), 231–59.

16. Charles Durrett, *Senior Cohousing: A Community Approach to Independent Living: The Handbook* (Berkeley: Habitat Press, 2005), 215.

17. Ibid., 215.

CHAPTER 3

1. Emily A. Greenfield, Andrew E. Scharlach, Carrie L. Graham, Joan K. Davitt, and Amanda J. Lehning, "A National Overview of Villages: Results from a 2012 Organizational Survey," Rutgers School of Social Work, December 1, 2012.

2. Leslie Marks, *Village Blueprint: Building a Community for All Ages* (Bethesda-Chevy Chase, MD: Bethesda-Chevy Chase Regional Services Center, 2010), *www.montgomerycountymd.gov.*

CHAPTER 4

1. Durrett, *Senior Cohousing,* 63.

2. Ibid., 16.

3. "Trailer Park as Community," Blaise Tobia to Cohousing-L mailing list, Feb. 17, 2010, *lists.cohousing.org/pipermail/cohousing-1.*

4. Durrett, *Senior Cohousing,* 54.

5. Ibid., 15, 19.

6. "Welcome to Takoma Village Cohousing," homepage, *www.takomavillage.org,* accessed Nov. 4, 2013.

7. Durrett, *Senior Cohousing,* 207.

8. David Wann, *Reinventing Community: Stories from the Walkways of Cohousing* (Golden CO: Fulcrum Publishing, 2005), 3.

9. "Consensus for Enduring Decisions Only," The Cohousing Association of the United States, *www.cohousing.org/cm/process/enduring.*

10. Durrett, *Senior Cohousing,* 72.

CHAPTER 5

1. *Profiles of a Movement: Co-operative Housing around the World* (Brussels: CECODHAS Housing Europe and ICA Housing, April 2012), 85, *www.housingeurope.eu/issue/2577.*

2. Richard Siegler and Herbert J. Levy, "Brief History of Cooperative Housing," *Cooperative Housing Journal* (1986): 12, *www.coophousing.org/uploadedFiles/NAHC_Site/Resources/nahc%20history%20Siegler.pdf.*

3. Ibid.

4. Ibid., 13.

5. "Cooperative Housing on the Lower East Side: A Brief History," Cooperative Village, accessed Dec. 17, 2013, *www.coopvillage.coop.*

6. Ibid.

7. "About Us: Not Just Bricks & Mortar," Penn South, last accessed Dec. 17, 2013, *www.pennsouth.coop/publicpages/about.html.*

8. Transportation may refer to cooperatives that have a bus, van, or driver for the community.

9. *Developing and Sustaining Rural Senior Cooperative Housing: Research Report* (Washington, DC: Cooperative Development Foundation, 2001), 9, *www.cdf. coop.*

10. Fred Wood, *Housing the Elderly: A Cooperative Partnership* (Warren, MI: CSI Support & Development Services, Sept. 9, 2005).

11. Gerry Glaser, "Housing Cooperatives for the Elderly," Presentation to the President's Commission on Housing, December 3, 1981, *www.seniorcoops.org/ glaser.html.*

12. "Housing List," Senior Cooperative Foundation, *www.seniorcoops.org/list.php.*

13. "Manufactured-home Cooperatives in NH," Community Loan Fund, *www. communityloanfund.org/how-we-help/roc-nh/nh-cooperatives.*

14. Richard (Dick) Martin, "A True Account of the History and Purchase of Green Pastures," *www.greenpasturesseniorcooperative.com.*

CHAPTER 6

1. Nat Yalowitz, *Penn South Program for Seniors: History of the First NORC Program in the United States* (New York: Penn South Social Services, Inc., 2011), 2.

2. Michael E. Hunt and Gail Gunter-Hunt, "Naturally Occurring Retirement Communities," *Journal of Housing for the Elderly* 3, no. 3–4 (1986), 3.

3. Ibid.

4. Yalowitz, *Growing Older,* 9.

5. Kristina L. Guo and Richard J. Castillo, "The U.S. Long Term Care System: Development and Expansion of Naturally Occurring Retirement Communities as an Innovative Model for Aging in Place," *Ageing International* 37 (2012): 219.

6. Bedney, Goldberg, and Josephson, "Aging in Place," 309.

7. See Community Innovations for Aging in Place Technical Assistance Resource Center, *www.ciaip.org.*

8. Guo and Castillo, "The U.S. Long Term Care System," 221.

9. Yalowitz, *Growing Older,* 11–12.

10. Yalowitz, *Penn South Program for Seniors,* 9.

11. Catharine Maclaren, Gerald Landsberg, and Harry Schwartz, "History, Accomplishments, Issues and Prospects of Supportive Service Programs in Naturally Occurring Retirement Communities in New York State: Lessons Learned," *Journal of Gerontological Social Work* 49, no. 1 (2007): 133.

12. Ibid.
13. Bedney, Goldberg, and Josephson, "Aging in Place," 312.
14. Guo and Castillo, "The U.S. Long Term Care System," 225.

CHAPTER 7

1. Victoria Bergman, "Elders Aging in Place: Princeton, New Jersey's Community Without Walls," Community Without Walls, Inc., 2000, *www.princetons.net/cww1/historyofCWW.html*.
2. Letter shared with author by Vicky Bergman, ©1992, 2012, CWW Inc.

CHAPTER 8

1. Wes Smith, *Hope Meadows: Real Life Stories of Healing and Caring from an Inspiring Community* (New York: Berkley Books, 2001), 179.

CHAPTER 9

1. MetLife Mature Market Institute, *2012 Market Survey of Long-Term Care Costs* (New York: MetLife Mature Market Institute, 2012), *www.metlife.com*.
2. Latisha R. Gray, "Assisted Living for RV Residents," *AARP,* June 14, 2010, *www.aarp.org*.
3. Tori Rodriguez, "Creativity Predicts a Longer Life," *Scientific American,* Sept. 9, 2012, *www.scientificamerican.com*.
4. Joan Jeffri, *Above Ground: Information on Artists III: Special Focus New York City Aging Artists* (New York: Columbia University/Research Center for Arts and Culture, 2007): 70, *artsandcultureresearch.org/Aging_artists*.
5. Gene D. Cohen, *The Mature Mind: The Power of the Aging Brain* (New York: Basic Books, 2005), 75–76.
6. *This American Life,* "Growth Spurt," Showtime, April 19, 2007.
7. Karen I. Fredriksen-Goldsen, et al., *The Aging and Health Report: Disparities and Resilience among Lesbian, Gay, Bisexual, and Transgender Older Adults* (Seattle: Institute for Multigenerational Health, 2011), 2, *www.caringandaging.org*.
8. Ibid., 38.
9. Ibid., 19.
10. *LGBT Older Adults in Long-Term Care Facilities: Stories from the Field* (Washington, DC: National Senior Citizens Law Center, 2011), *www.nsclc.org*.
11. MetLife Mature Market Institute, *Still Out, Still Aging: The MetLife Study of Lesbian, Gay, Bisexual, and Transgender Baby Boomers* (New York: MetLife Mature Market Institute, March 2010), 17, *www.metlife.com*.
12. "Outdoor Recreation," Birds of a Feather Resort Community, last accessed Dec. 12, 2013, *birdsofafeather.com/index.php?page=outdoor-recreation*.

CHAPTER 10

1. Laryssa Mykytta and Suzanne Macartney, *Sharing a Household: Composition and Economic Well-Being: 2007–2010* (Washington, DC: US Census Bureau, 2012), *www.census.gov*.

2. Louise S. Machinist, Jean McQuillin, and Karen M. Bush, *My House, Our House: Living Far Better for Far Less in a Cooperative Household* (Pittsburgh: St. Lynn's Press, 2013), 95.

3. Tatjana Meschede, Thomas M. Shapiro, and Jennifer Wheary, *Living Longer on Less: The New Economic (In)Security of Seniors* (Waltham, MA: The Institute on Assets and Social Policy and Dēmos, 2009), 1-2, *www.demos.org*.

4. Federal Interagency Forum on Aging-Related Statistics, *Older Americans 2012: Key Indicators of Well-Being* (Washington, DC: US Government Printing Office, June 2012), 21–22, *agingstats.gov*.

5. Barry L. Steffen, et al., *Worst Case Housing Needs 2009: Report to Congress* (Washington, DC: US Department of Housing and Urban Development Office of Policy Development and Outreach, Feb. 2011), 5, *www.huduser.org*.

6. George C. Hemmens, Charles J. Hoch, and Jana Carp, eds., *Under One Roof: Issues and Innovations in Shared Housing* (Albany: State University of New York Press, 1996), 6.

CHAPTER 11

1. Robin McKee, "Wisdom of Grandparents Helped Rise of Prehistoric Man," *The Guardian Observer,* July 23, 2011, *www.guardian.co.uk/science/2011/jul/24/prehistoric-man-helped-as-elderly-survived*.

2. Pew Research Center, *The Return of the Multigenerational Family Household: A Social and Demographic Trends Report* (Washington, DC: Pew Research Center, March 18, 2010), 4, *www.pewsocialtrends.org/files/2010/10/752-multi-generational-families.pdf*.

3. Generations United, *Family Matters: Multigenerational Households in a Volatile Economy* (Washington, DC: Generations United, 2011), 1, *www.gu.org*.

4. Ibid., 6.

5. Pew Research Center, *The Return of the Multigenerational Family Household,* 7.

6. MetLife Mature Market Institute, *Multigenerational Views on Family Financial Obligations* (New York: MetLife Mature Market Institute, January 2012), 15, *www.metlife.com*.

7. MetLife Mature Market Institute, *Grandparents Investing in Grandchildren: A MetLife Study on how Grandparents Share their Time, Values, and Money* (New York: MetLife Mature Market Institute, September 2012), 5, *www.metlife.com*.

8. MetLife Mature Market Institute, *Grandparents Investing,* 4.

CHAPTER 12

1. National Council on Aging, *Falls Prevention: Fact Sheet* (Washington, DC: National Council on Aging, 2012), *www.ncoa.org*.

2. Australian Ageing Agenda, "All New Homes to be 'Livable' by 2020," July 15, 2010, *www.australianageingagenda.com.au*.

3. Penelope Green, "Under One Roof, Building for Extended Families," *New York Times,* Nov. 29, 2012, 1, *www.nytimes.com*.

4. Matthew Heimer, "Pitching 'Granny Pods' to Aging Parents," *Encore* (blog), *Wall Street Journal Market Watch,* Nov. 28, 2012, *blogs.marketwatch.com/encore.*

5. Fredrick Kunkle, "Pioneering the Granny Pod: Fairfax County Family Adapts to High-Tech Dwelling that Could Change Elder Care," *Washington Post,* Nov. 25, 2012, *www.washingtonpost.com.*

6. Cara Bailey Fausset, Andrew J. Kelly, Wendy A. Rogers, and Arthur D. Fisk, "Challenges to Aging in Place: Understanding Home Maintenance Difficulties," *Journal of Housing for the Elderly* 25, no. 2 (Spring 2011), 125–141, *www.ncbi. nlm.nih.gov/pmc/articles.*

7. *The Maturing of America: Communities Moving Forward for an Aging Population* (Washington, DC: National Association of Area Agencies on Aging, June 2011), i, *www.n4a.org.*

8. To view short videos of Lifelong Mableton's vision, visit *www. theagingamericaproject.com/video_where-we-live.php.*

9. Philadelphia Corporation for Aging, *Laying the Foundation for an Age-Friendly Philadelphia: A Progress Report* (Philadelphia: Philadelphia Corporation for Aging, June 2011), *www.pcacares.org/Files/PCA_Age-Friendly_WhitePaper_web. pdf.*

CHAPTER 13

1. MetLife Mature Market Institute, *MetLife Long-Term Care IQ: Removing Myths, Reinforcing Realities* (New York: MetLife Mature Market Institute, September 2009), 5, *www.metlife.com.*

2. Sara Mansfield Taber, "Caring for Mom, Mum and Maman," *Washington Post,* January 10, 2010, *www.washingtonpost.com.*

3. Families USA Foundation, *Cutting Medicaid: Harming Seniors and People with Disabilities Who Need Long-Term Care* (Washington, DC: Families USA, May 2011), 2, *www.familiesusa.org.*

4. Kaiser Commission on Medicaid and the Uninsured, *State Options that Expand Access to Medicaid Home and Community-Based Services* (Washington, DC: Henry J. Kaiser Family Foundation, Oct. 2011), 5, *www.kff.org.*

5. American Association of Homes and Services for the Aging [now called Leading Age], *In a Place They Call Home: Expanding Consumer Choice through Home and Community-Based Services* (Washington, DC: American Association of Homes and Services for the Aging, Jan. 2009), 7–8, *www.hospitalathome.org/files/ HCBS_Cabinet_Report_Final-PDF_version.pdf.*

6. Ibid., 9.

7. Ari Houser, *Insight on the Issues: A New Way of Looking at Private Pay Affordability of Long-Term Services and Supports* (Washington, DC: AARP Public Policy Institute, Oct. 2012), 1, *www.aarp.org.*

8. Lynn Feinberg, Susan C. Reinhard, Ari Houser, and Rita Choula, *Valuing the Invaluable: 2011 Update—The Growing Contributions and Costs of Family Caregiving* (Washington, DC: AARP Public Policy Institute, 2011), 3, *www. aarp.org.*

9. Ari Houser, Mary Jo Gibson, and Donald L. Redfoot, *Trends in Family Caregiving and Paid Home Care for Older People with Disabilities in the Community: Data from the National Long-Term Care Survey* (Washington, DC: AARP Public Policy Institute, Sept. 2010), 4, *www.aarp.org.*

10. Robert H. Binstock, "Resource Allocation in an Aging Society," in *Public Health for an Aging Society,* ed. Thomas R. Prohaska, Lynda A. Anderson, Robert H. Binstock (Baltimore: Johns Hopkins University Press, 2012), 404.

11. Eileen J. Tell and Nancy P. Morith, "Long-Term Care Insurance: Benefits, Costs, Options," *Public Policy & Aging Report* 23, no. 1 (Winter 2013), 18–19.

12. David Segal, "A Winding Road to Benefits from Long-Term Care Insurance," *New York Times,* March 24, 2013, *www.nytimes.com.*

13. Jessica S. Miller, Xiaomei Shi, and Marc A. Cohen, *Private Long-Term Care Insurance: Following an Admission Cohort over 28 Months to Track Claim Experience, Service Use and Transitions* (Washington, DC: US Department of Health and Human Services, April 2008), *aspe.hhs.gov.*

14. MetLife Mature Market Institute, *MetLife Long-Term Care IQ,* 6. See also T. Tompson, et al., *Long-Term Care: Perceptions, Experiences, and Attitudes among Americans 40 or Older (Final Report)* (Chicago: The Associated Press-NORC Center for Public Affairs Research, 2013), *www.apnorc.org/projects.*

15. "Who Needs Care?" US Department of Health and Human Services, *longtermcare.gov/the-basics/who-needs-care.*

16. Tell and Morith, "Long-Term Care Insurance," 21.

17. Barbara R. Stucki, "New Directions for Policy and Research on Reverse Mortgages," *Public Policy & Aging Report* 23, no. 1 (2013): 12.

CHAPTER 14

1. Paraprofessional Healthcare Institute, *Facts 3: America's Direct Care Workforce* (November 2013 Update), (Bronx, NY: Paraprofessional Healthcare Institute, 2013) *phinational.org/sites/phinational.org/files/phi-facts-3.pdf.*

2. Bureau of Labor Statistics, U.S. Department of Labor, *Occupational Outlook Handbook,* 2012–13 Edition, Home Health and Personal Care Aides, on the Internet at *www.bls.gov/ooh/healthcare/home-health-and-personal-care-aides.htm.*

3. Bureau of Labor Statistics, *Occupational Outlook Handbook,* "Work Environment."

4. Paraprofessional Healthcare Institute, *Facts 3,* 4.

5. Ibid.

6. Walter Leutz, "Foreign-Born Workers in Long-Term Supportive Services," *Public Policy & Aging Report* 22, no. 2 (April 2012): 17–18.

7. Committee on the Future Health Care Workforce for Older Americans, *Retooling for an Aging America: Building the Health Care Workforce* (Washington, DC: Institute of Medicine, April 2008), 9, *www.iom.edu/Reports/2008/Retooling-for-an-aging-America-Building-the-Health-Care-Workforce.aspx.*

8. Ibid., 29.

9. Brian K. Unwin and Paul E. Tatum, III, "House Calls," *American Family Physician* 83, no. 8 (2011): 925–31.
10. Lesley Cryer, Scott B. Shannon, Melanie Van Amsterdam, and Bruce Leff, "Costs for 'Hospital at Home' Patients Were 19 Percent Lower, with Equal or Better Outcomes Compared to Similar Inpatients," *Health Affairs* 31, no. 6 (June 2012): 1237.
11. Stacy Dale, Randall Brown, Barbara Lepidus Carlson, "How Do Hired Workers Fare under Consumer-Directed Personal Care," *The Gerontologist* 45, no. 5 (2005): 583.

CHAPTER 15

1. *Robot & Frank*, directed by Jake Schreier (2012; Culver City, CA: Sony Pictures Home Entertainment, 2013), DVD.
2. Cory-Ann Smarr, et al., "Older Adults' Preferences for and Acceptance of Robot Assistance for Everyday Living Tasks," *Proceedings of the Human Factors and Ergonomics Society 56th Annual Meeting-2012*, Boston, MA, 153.
3. To view videos of PR2 in action, visit Willow Garage's website *www.willowgarage.com*.
4. M. R. Banks, L. M. Willoughby, and W. A. Banks, "Animal-Assisted Therapy and Loneliness in Nursing Homes: Use of Robotic Versus Living Dogs," *Journal of American Medical Directors Association* 9, no. 3 (2008): 173–77.
5. Jiska Cohen-Mansfield, et al., "The Value of Social Attributes of Stimuli for Promoting Engagement in Persons With Dementia," *Journal of Nervous and Mental Disorders* 198, no. 8 (2010): 586–92. *www.ncbi.nlm.nih.gov/pmc*.
6. Jacob Shatzer, "Are We Forming Ourselves for a Posthuman Future?," *Ethics & Medicine* 28 no. 2 (July 1, 2012): 81.
7. Linda L. Barrett, *Healthy@Home 2.0* (Washington, DC: AARP Research and Strategic Analysis, April 2011), 1, *www.aarp.org*.
8. Andrew Broderick and David Lindeman, *Scaling Telehealth Programs: Lessons from Early Adopters* (pub. 1654) (New York: The Commonwealth Fund, Jan. 2013), *www.commonwealthfund.org/Publications/Case-Studies/2013/Jan/Telehealth-Synthesis.aspx*.
9. Kathryn Zickuhr and Mary Madden, *Older Adults and Internet Use* (Washington, DC: Pew Research Center, June 6, 2012), *www.pewinternet.org*.
10. Laurie M. Orlov, *Technology for Aging in Place: 2013 Market Overview* (Aging in Place Technology Watch, July 2013), 11, *www.ageinplacetech.com*.
11. Sara E. McBride, et al., "Challenges of Training Older Adults in a Home Health Care Context," *Proceedings of the Human Factors and Ergonomics Society 56th Annual Meeting-2012*, Boston, MA, 2492.
12. Sara E. McBride, Jenay M. Beer, Tracy L. Mitzner, & Wendy A. Rogers, "Challenges for Home Health Care Providers: A Needs Assessment," *Physical & Occupational Therapy in Geriatrics* 29, no. 1 (2011): 17.
13. University of Ulster, "Ulster Research To Develop Hi-Tech Clothing For

Elderly," June 1, 2009, *news.ulster.ac.uk/releases/2009/4420.html.*

14. Ruth Dempsey, "Interview with Maggie Mort: The Trouble with Telecare," *Aging Horizons Bulletin,* March/April 2013, *aginghorizons.com.*

15. Maggie Mort, Celia Roberts, and Blanca Callén, "Ageing with Telecare: Care or Coercion in Austerity?," *Sociology of Health & Illness* 20, no. 10 (2012): 1–4.

16. Dempsey, "Interview with Maggie Mort."

CHAPTER 16

1. Allan S. Teel, *Alone and Invisible No More—How Grassroots Community Action and 21st Century Technologies Can Empower Elders to Stay in Their Homes and Lead Healthier, Happier Lives* (White River Junction: Chelsea Green Publishing, 2011), 29.

2. Genworth, *Genworth 2013 Cost of Care Survey: Home Care Providers, Adult Day Health Care Facilities, Assisted Living Facilities and Nursing Homes* (New York: Genworth Life Insurance Company, 2013), *www.genworth.com.*

3. Charlene Harrington, Helen Carrillo, and Brandee Woleslagle Blank, *Nursing Facilities, Staffing, Residents and Facility Deficiencies, 2003 through 2008* (San Francisco: Dept. of Social and Behavioral Sciences, University of California, Nov. 2009), 72, *www.theconsumervoice.org.*

4. Ibid., 2.

5. National PACE Association, "What is PACE: List of PACE Programs by State." See a list of locations at *www.npaonline.org.*

6. Stephanie Bouchard, "Disruptive Innovators: Structured Family Caregiving," *Healthcare Finance News,* March 2013, *www.healthcarefinancenews.com.*

Index